BRAIN INJURY TRAUMA AND GRIEF

ADDITIONAL TITLES BY SHIREEN JEEJEEBHOY

Lifeliner: The Judy Taylor Story
The Job Sessions: Why Do The Innocent Suffer?
She
Eleven Shorts +1
Concussion Is Brain Injury
Aban's Accension
Time and Space
Concussion Is Brain Injury: Treating the Neurons and Me
Louise and The Men of Transit

ONLINE PRESENCE

Twitter @ShireenJ
jeejeebhoy.ca
psychologytoday.com/ca/blog/concussion-is-brain-injury
concussionisbraininjury.com
concussionisbraininjury.ca
Facebook: Shireen Jeejeebhoy
Flickr: flickr.com/photos/pario/
LinkedIn: Shireen Jeejeebhoy

PRAISE

"Jeejeebhoy is a passionate advocate for patients, and a sympathetic narrator."
– SPR on Concussion Is Brain Injury: Treating the Neurons and Me

"Put simply this is the best urban fantasy story that I have ever read period."
– Shane Porteous, Writer, gives She 5 stars on Smashwords

"A compelling story....Reading [Lifeliner] will make you laugh, smile, cringe, cry and most importantly, think."
– Diana Rohini LaVigne, Online Editor, Indian Life & Style Magazine

"What an amazing journey into the future!"
– Ana on Time and Space on Goodreads

BRAIN INJURY, TRAUMA, AND GRIEF

HOW TO HEAL WHEN YOU ARE ALONE

Shireen Anne Jeejeebhoy

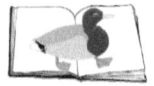

Copyright © 2022 Shireen Anne Jeejeebhoy

All rights reserved.

No part of this publication may be reproduced, stored in a retrieval system or transmitted, in any form or by any means, electronic, mechanical, recording or otherwise (except brief passages for purposes of review) without the prior permission of the author or a licence from The Canadian Copyright Licensing Agency (Access Copyright). For an Access Copyright licence, visit www.accesscopyright.ca or call toll free to 1-800-893-5777.

Cover Design and Illustrations by and copyright © 2022 Shireen Anne Jeejeebhoy

Cover fonts Exodus Standard and Exodus Display by Andrew Herndon, under Commercial License.

Interior fonts Montserrat by The Montserrat Project Authors and Cormorant by Christian Thalmann, Principal Designer, both licenced under the Open Font License.

Scripture quotations contained herein are either from the New Revised Standard Version Bible, copyright © 1989, by the Division of Christian Education of the National Council of the Churches of Christ in the U.S.A., and are used by permission. All rights reserved; Or from The Holy Bible, New International Version® NIV® Copyright © 1973, 1978, 1984, 2011 by Biblica, Inc. Used with permission. All rights reserved worldwide.

Licence Notes, Print Edition

This book is licenced for your personal enjoyment only. This book may not be resold or given away to other people. If you would like to share this book with another person, please purchase an additional copy for each recipient. If you're reading this book and did not purchase it, or it was not purchased for your use only, then please return and purchase your own copy. Thank you for respecting the hard work of this author.

First Printing, 2022

ISBN-978-1-7753514-9-8

To the Prolifiko writing community

*And to Mum and Dad,
who persevered through leaving ancestral homes,
difficulties and upheaval,
to create successful lives together*

Table of Contents

Welcome 1
1   Purpose 7

STEP ZERO: PREPARATION

2   Deep Breathing 12
3   Tools 15
4   Pre-Injury Stress Busters 23
5   Today's Stress Busters 28
6   Time 39

STEP ONE: LOVED AND UNLOVED

7   A New Word: Mithra! 48
8   God or Nature 53
9   What Is Relationship? 57
10 Recipient of Love 68
11 Unloved 75
12 Unexplainable Encounters 85
13 How Do We Get To Feeling Worthy of Life? 90

STEP TWO: RELATIONSHIPS

14 Relationship With Ourself 96
15 Relationships With Others 109
16 Book of Job on Friendships 122
17 Forgiveness Is Not Reconciliation 129

STEP THREE: GRIEF

18 Definitions 150
19 Acknowledge Losses 156
20 Regrets 184
21 Trauma 189

STEP FOUR: HEALING GRIEF

22 You Are Not The Injury... 196
23 Action Plan: Saying Au Revoir to You......................... 204

STEP FIVE: TREATING YOUR NEURONS

24 Brain-Based Understanding... 220
25 Lessons I've Learned... 224
26 Emotional Courage 240
27 Neurostimulation Therapies Work................................ 256
28 Treating Your Neurons 261
29 Stretching Your Connections 271
Readings... 283
Acknowledgements 288

WELCOME

Welcome to the world of brain injury, an unimaginable world. A world you and I don't want to be in. And definitely not alone in it! I used to ask myself, "How on earth did this happen?! This isn't the future I envisioned!" How many times have we heard about self-fulfilling prophecies and needing to visualize the future we want? I've lost count. It's so frustrating because I certainly didn't prophesy brain injury. After brain injury, you might as well visualize teleporting onto the Enterprise deck with Captain Kirk, for all visualizing doesn't work. Brain injury, trauma, and grief throw up sky-high, Earth-thick barriers. You can visualize the future you want until the stars plummet into the ocean, but until you're treating the neurons and healing the trauma and brain injury grief, visualizing ain't gonna work.

But make no mistake, you in all your brain injury glory, sunk in the pain of trauma and grief, are an integral part of the universe. A unique, desired light. The universe wants you here, heard your pained cry to heal, and led you to this book to demolish those barriers. Once you've treated your neurons, faced your trauma, and begun healing brain injury grief, then you can visualize the person you want to be.

When I gave up visualizing and shed the guilt of self-fulfilling prophecy talk, I wrote. Writing connects me with you and eases the aloneness.

I began my brain injury writings with my memoir *Concussion Is Brain Injury*. I revised it substantially five years later, subtitling it, "Treating the Neurons and Me." That netted me an invitation to write a blog on brain injury for *Psychology Today*. Then when the pandemic hit, it freed up enough of my energy to create a website on what brain injury is, appropriate diagnostics, and effective treatments. But one piece remained missing: healing the grief and finding the wherewithal to pursue treatments that heal. The medical system does neither. I hope this book will fill in that gap, make you feel connected with others in this world and less alone, and give you the emotional courage to go forth and find treatments that will regenerate your broken neurons. May these three resources of memoir, brain injury website, and this book help you find a life you love.

What Is Brain Injury? A Synopsis.

Brain injury can happen from any cause that damages brain tissue. Since the brain controls everything, anything and everything can be injured.

What does that include? In a nutshell, brain injury can disrupt your mobility, emotions, thinking, speaking and listening, anger, body's metabolism, etc. etc.

Neurons

Neurons are the basic cells that make up our brain. Bundled together, they form neural networks. Neurons talk to each other to make the brain function. No talking, no function. An axon, like an electrical wire, connects the two ends of a neuron. Electrical impulses pulse down the axon and tell the neuron's Medusa end to stream out neurotransmitters. Adjacent neurons receive those neurotransmitters, which trigger a pulse down the next neurons' axons. That is how they communicate. Some axons are short; long ones cross the brain from one side to another. They likely connect far-apart functions like hearing with thinking.

Then an injury happens; those long axons break; suddenly those far-apart areas become deaf to each other. Hearing a sentence, for example, doesn't lead to immediate thought about it. Instead, thought appears after the ears pulse the message through a roundabout route of neurons with shorter axons. Like a slow telephone tag. Things get a little mixed up taking that slower route. To regain immediate thought, the brain has to regrow those longer axons and regenerate dead and broken neurons. But how?

WELCOME

Microglia

Microglia are cute little cells that maintain neurons, keeping them humming those pulses along their axons. They ensure neurotransmitters stream out and are received by the next neurons in the neural network. They also sweep out bad proteins and eat detritus. Frankly, I couldn't figure out what happened to what they eat. Does it get pooped out? Turned into energy? My research didn't turn up a straightforward explanation about their micro-digestive systems when they gobble up what they see as trash.

When an injury happens, microglia turn mean. They spot injured neurons, scream there's trash there, and eat them. Then they tell their fellow microglia in uninjured parts of the brain, "You'd better eat those neurons!" And they do! That's how brain injury worsens over days and weeks. They call this worsening "secondary" or "cascading injury."

As part of the immune system, microglia also turn mean when a virus enters the body. Evolutionarily, microglia's job is to make you lethargic and take to your bed so you don't spread the virus to other people.

When your immune system defeats the virus, microglia transform back to happy neuron supporters, and you get up off your bed.

With brain injury, though, the microglia need a nudge to stop being mean and to regenerate neurons. Yes, the brain can regenerate, and microglia are an essential part of that feature. Neurostimulation and neuromodulation therapies reboot microglia back to being neuron supporters and accelerate the brain's regeneration, including regrowing those long axons.

LEARN MORE

> "Brain injury is not a single event, but a process over time initiated by an event. The injury becomes the sum of the cause plus the hidden cascading damage after." Read about the neuroscience behind brain injury, with references and videos, at https://concussionisbraininjury.com/education/what-is-brain-injury/.

Depression After Brain Injury Is Not a Mood Disorder

Let's take depression as an example of one brain injury symptom, since it's such a common "diagnosis" after brain injury.

Depression involves part of the frontal lobe. It can emerge when injury damages neurons in those areas. Neurons in snooze mode make you look kind of down. Then microglia turn mean. The microglia make you lethargic so that your body uses all its resources to fight off the invader (the injury) while protecting members of your community from the culprit in case it's contagious. They eat up dead neurons and stop sweeping out bad proteins and keeping healthy neurons healthy. They instruct microglia in uninjured parts of your brain to eat their neurons, and you take longer naps.

Then your situation worsens. You never expected your life to take a sudden turn for the worse. It's all too much. Situational depression affects people with brain injury, too. Improve the situation, and like magic, depression lifts!

Depression here is not a mood disorder—it's a combination of injured neurons no longer keeping your emotions and thinking on a healthy plane, microglia sending you to bed, and your situation becoming overwhelming. Medications flooding your brain with neurotransmitters may flatten your mood or temporarily give you enough energy to make your bed, but they don't restore neurons or regrow axons. They don't tell microglia to stop being mean and start supporting your neurons again. They also don't improve your situation.

Don't stop your anti-depressants on your own before embarking on neurostimulation therapies under medical guidance!

What you need to treat depression after brain injury is therapies that reboot microglia, regenerate neurons, and regrow the long axons, as well as social and health support to change your situation from overwhelming to cope-able.

Brain Injury Anger Needs Treating Not Management

The same principle applies to anything brain injury changed in you such as brain injury anger, the anger that flashes on out of the blue and vanishes as suddenly and shocks everyone, including yourself, when it does. Strategies don't work well; anger management is the wrong treatment; being blamed worsens your feelings of self-worth and exacerbates your injury. Treating the injury, believe it or not, heals brain injury anger by first vanquishing the nails-on-chalkboard irritation from overload then restoring healthy function to those areas of the brain involved in emotions, sensory function, social communication, and anger control. And probably more areas than that because we still don't fully understand the neurophysiological basis of anger.

Remember: anger is foremost a self-protective mechanism. Perhaps brain injury anger both tells you and those around you you're being overloaded and takes you out of a situation your brain literally cannot process. With all those dead neurons and broken axons and microglia busily eating them up, how can your brain process anything in the way it used to?

Personality

When I studied psychology, the Diagnostic and Statistical Manual of Mental Disorders or DSM was in its third iteration. Growing up in the medical world biased my view toward seeing the DSM as exciting, innovative, and scientific, unlike what had come before in our understanding of mental illness. I chewed over what my psychology professors taught: labels limit people so avoid them. But I thought the DSM labels informed rather than bound—except for what they called, "personality disorders."

I questioned how can a personality be disordered? A personality is who you are. We can see a personality easily, yet trying to describe its scientific or brain basis stumps us. We can talk about what comprises personality, but even now we're only guessing. Philosophers and psychologists, pastors and lay people, ill and healthy, think about personality from their own perspectives. I found that after brain injury, my concept of personality underwent a profound change. My injury had killed so much of myself and hid what remained. That led to me questioning my identity: what is identity, what is personality?

I returned to the puzzling concept of personality disorder. Perhaps what is disordered is the *manifestation* of personality; the personality itself is not disordered. But asking myself, "How does personality manifest itself?" backtracked me to the DSM category of personality disorders. I thought, *We need to know what personality is before we can talk about it.*

We don't know what personality is.

Steeped in the intellectual and medical science world from birth on, I know scientists and intellectuals are very good at rationalizing the indefensible and have no trouble using words to make rubbish research sound groundbreaking. So when they talk about personality as if it's known, they're using the same rationalizing skills.

We don't know exactly where personality exists in the brain.

What I know is we all have a good personality,* but a brain injury locks away a person's original personality. The physical trauma alters our brain activity and distorts and binds aspects of our personality. These changes create both grief and a search for identity and new purpose. Treating the neurons and healing trauma can resurrect parts, or perhaps all, of our original personality.

A Good Personality

You have a good personality. Brain dysfunction, illness, or injury is not personality. No matter how much brain injury has vanished your good personality or distorted your emotions or slowed your thoughts down to frozen molasses speed, you have a good personality. Just because you don't know who you are, others don't see you as "good" anymore, and psychiatry labels you with a mood, attention, memory, or personality disorder, doesn't change the fact you have a good personality.

Combine this knowledge with knowing God loves you and Nature created you to be an intrinsic and valuable part, and use it to energize your way to healing your brain. Reject the labels that bind you into ill health and keep you stuck in untreated brain injury and trauma. Climb off the useless treadmill of strategies and rest *as treatment* and instead pursue treating your injured neurons and healing your trauma and brain injury grief.

Treating your neurons may never get rid of the need for rest and naps, but it will diminish them. As your neurons regrow and reconnect under the power of neurostimulation, strategies mostly will become what chaining the mentally ill to walls became: obsolete. And you'll heal your identity and find your purpose.

---

*I won't deny evil people exist at the most ordinary levels of our lives. But they are few. What makes them troubling is how much influence they can wield, how so many gravitate towards and elevate them instead of spotting them for who they are and avoiding them. Good people do bad things, but that doesn't make them evil. And so though the word "all" is a generalization, it's one rooted in reality.

CHAPTER 1

PURPOSE

When I Was Eleven

I stood in the sliding glass doorway of my grandfather's cardiac care unit room. He lay white and still surrounded by humming machines and tubes in the hushed room. My father had gotten special permission for me to visit him. Back then, hospitals allowed only those fourteen and older to visit patients. I was eleven.

My grandfather croaked, "Hello." We stood around him, and in that moment, I wanted to help him heal. As an eleven-year-old, I knew only doctors can heal people.

As we left, I saw through the glass walls and glass doors of another room, a young man lying in his bed alone, no visitors. I felt his loneliness and fear. I thought, *Children have their parents and families to comfort them in their fear, but who do adults have?* Adults need as much comforting as children. Why do we pretend otherwise?

Who Will Comfort the Adults?

Decades later, I entered the hellscape of brain injury. My closed head injury, aka concussion, caused many losses. But I think the most destructive one was the loss of innocence. Innocence in my trust and beliefs. I lost trust in loved ones to be there through hard years, to support and help me find treatments to heal my injured neurons. I lost trust in physicians, psychiatrists, and neurologists to learn and do all they can to help me achieve full recovery. I lost the belief that my life was worth saving. I stopped believing medicine would treat me the same under brain injury care as under all other medical specialties. Health care professionals treated my injury unhurriedly, as if I have nothing to offer society unlike everyone else. Most profoundly, losing my reading and being abandoned, something unimaginable before the brain injury, rocked me like I'd unwittingly stepped on a bomb and had no parachute to land on sturdy ground.

This book is for you, who, like me, have lost innocence and experienced abandonment. You who find the grind of your reality almost beyond enduring yet don't know how to get hold of treatments that'll heal your injured neurons.

A Caution

Do not stop any of your medications on your own, especially anti-seizure or epilepsy medications! Stopping medications that act on the brain can lead to catastrophic consequences and should only be done under medical supervision. And definitely **not before** embarking on neurostimulation therapies, but **only alongside or afterwards under medical supervision**. Responsible practitioners of neurostimulation and neuromodulation therapies work with your prescriber to gently, carefully, under strict, careful guidance decrease or take you off medication when and as it's safe and appropriate to do so. You don't want to worsen your brain injury by prematurely coming off your medications, right? You want to make it better. I hope this book will help you embark on the road to doing that.

As always, confer with your trusted medical or psychological health provider, as medical and health-care-related information provided herein, in the absence of a visit with a health-care professional, must be

Purpose

considered as an educational service only. This book is not designed to replace a physician's independent judgement about the appropriateness or risks of a procedure or therapy for a given patient or client. The purpose of this book is to provide you with information that will help you make your own health-care decisions. The information and opinions provided here are believed to be accurate and sound, based on the best judgement available to the author, editors, and publisher. Readers who fail to consult appropriate health authorities assume the risk of any injuries. The publisher and author are not responsible for errors or omissions. The editors and publisher welcome any reader to report to the publisher any discrepancies or inaccuracies noticed..

Step Zero

PREPARATION

CHAPTER 2
———

DEEP BREATHING

To heal brain injury, trauma, and grief, we must acquire basic tools to support us through the pain that healing brings. The difference between the pain of loneliness, injury, anxiety, and fear that your situation is forever and the pain of healing is that the latter diminishes as you walk that path. The former may hide out for a while until sadness erupts like a massive volcano and blankets you in the ash of grief.

The first and most basic tool my psychologist taught me was deep breathing.

deep breathing for two minutes calms your nervous system →

By expanding your respiratory muscles and increasing air flow, deep breathing counters stress. It won't rid you of anxiety induced by neurons chaotically vibrating and probably won't lower your resting heart rate from triple digits, but it will give you a focus and help settle you during stressful moments.

Practice deep breathing in a quiet room by yourself. I had to practice for months before it became automatic. But it's worth it.

How to Deep Breathe

Deep breathing sounds simple. Inhale and exhale. How hard is that? We all know how to breathe! But good deep breathing follows a sine curve. A gentle rise, a pause at the top, a gentler slope down, and another pause before the curve of your breathing rises again, as like mine, shown below.

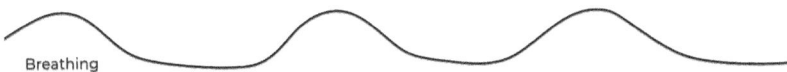
Breathing

You aim for about six breaths a minute without becoming dizzy, although you may experience dizziness the first few tries. Perhaps you'll start at eight breaths per minute or ten or twelve. With practice, you'll progress it down to six. Use an app that will count the seconds for you and calculate your breathing rate.

Put one hand on your stomach and expand it against your hand as you inhale. Feeling the expansion is a physical reminder to inhale deep into your lungs. Feeling the movement through your hand also relaxes and assures you you're doing it right. Count up from one as you breathe in and the same number as you breathe out.

Apps and devices that measure your heart rate as you deep breathe will give you feedback on your heart rate variability and whether you're boosting your physiology.

A Note on Heart Rate Variability

Heart rate variability (HRV) is a measure of how well your heart rate rises and falls in sync with your inhalations and exhalations. The higher the HRV, the better the synchronization between the two. After brain injury, your heart rate may be erratic like mine. That leads to a low HRV. Seen on a computer screen, good HRV looks like two smooth curves rising and falling in sync, similar to mine as shown below.

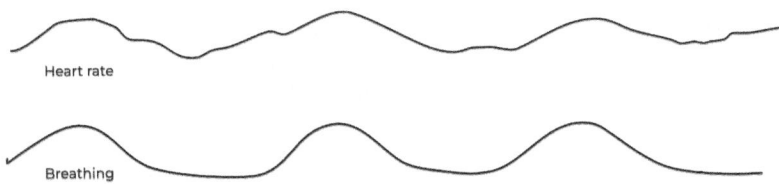
Heart rate

Breathing

With low HRV, the heart rate bucks like sharp waves, surging and plunging erratically (see below). Yet deep breathing can still settle the nerves. Practicing it meant I'd start deep breathing automatically when under pressure. I mayn't be able to control my resting heart rate with it nor increase my HRV, but I can use it to focus on and temporarily steady my breathing and heart rate during stressful encounters. Being realistic about what deep breathing can do avoids frustration and abandoning it altogether.

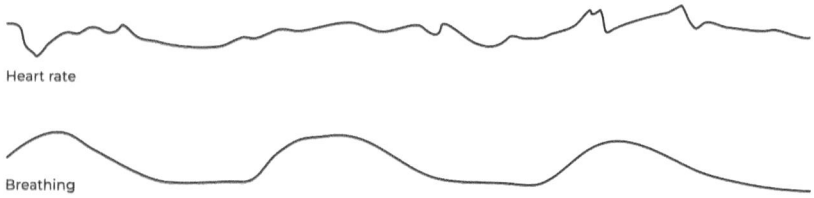

Heart rate

Breathing

LEARN MORE

> Photobiomodulation (low-intensity laser) and gamma brainwave enhancement therapies began my heart rate to synchronize with my breathing and inch my HRV upward. See https://concussionisbraininjury.com/treatments for more information on these therapies.

When to Deep Breathe

Practice deep breathing a couple of minutes to start, then increasing to five minutes, using an app and/or video to guide you.

Once you've mastered deep breathing in a quiet room on your own, start practicing it when you're with a friendly person like your favourite health care provider, then moving on to situations when your brain struggles to cope like with that judgemental family member we all have.

Each time you sit down to read this book, begin your session with deep breathing for two minutes, even if you don't feel you've mastered it. That'll be part of your practice. And if you've reached automaticity in your practice, continue deep breathing as you read. Healing is stressful; deep breathing is a basic tool to help you navigate that stress.

CHAPTER 3

TOOLS

Paper, Ink, and Digital

Pen and Paper

The next step in preparing to read this book is to gather notebooks, highlighters, and pens or pencils. I buy my notebooks and pens in bulk. I collect markers and highlighters in pinks, purples, yellows, and blues, colours that let me be playful while working.

Some self-help books include a space for writing in, but I find it's never enough for me. Perhaps I'm too wordy or my writing is too big and loopy to fit the space. Cheap Hilroy notebooks, like the ones we used in school, work well. They have spiral bindings that lay flat. On the other hand, beautiful notebooks like the ones by paperblank remind you that you're worth the work and healing is beautiful. If you're limited in funds, consider decorating your notebook pages and covers instead. Buy coloured pencils to draw with as you follow the Action Plans. Don't think; let your subconscious work through your fingers.

Title the first notebook "Stress and Grieving," the second notebook "Stories for Healing," the third one "Relationships," and the fourth one "Hello Healing."

Playing in Ink

As adults, we don't play enough. Your brain injury has become a grinding job. Rebel! Give yourself permission to spend your money and energy on the tools of healing. Even if you can't afford expensive paperblank notebooks, find a fountain pen. Today, you can buy fountain pens for $5.00 and ink cartridges in many colours. Buy a couple of these pens and two different ink colours. Each colour can represent something that's important to you or can simply add a playful element as you work through the Action Plans. Let your subconscious choose the colours of the pens and the inks.

Stickers

Fun or pretty or favourite stickers add a rewarding note. Place a sticker next to each Action Plan or step you've done or to highlight a point you want to return to. But highlight sparingly. Otherwise, the stickers will become a mess and nothing will stand out.

A Note on Digital

You may prefer to use digital notebooks on your tablet or laptop. In that case, try to use styluses to check off completed actions or star partially completed actions. Choose different colours for your stylus "ink."

ePaper, such as the latest ReMarkable, has both the feel of writing on paper with pen, pencil, or marker along with the advantages of digital, such as working in the cloud on different devices, typing or handwriting, and search capability.

Journals

If you aren't journalling, start. Buy a bunch of lined journals that appeal to you and pens that are easy to write with. You're more likely to use journals you like and to write with pens that don't drain your energy, or at least not too much, than if you buy utilitarian tools you don't like.

Journalling is where you'll:
- Write down your thoughts and feelings, or what you want to feel but cannot.
- Record events from a few days ago you're now processing.
- Document confusing social encounters and daily happenings.
- Capture the day with nightly writing before your memory fades.

Handwrite in Physical Journals

Even if you use digital notebooks for the Action Plans, it's important to handwrite in your journals. Handwriting connects a different part of your brain than typing. The tactile feel of paper, the practice of holding a pen and coordinating your eyes and hands to write, will help heal some of your finer motor functions, as well. Even if your fine motor skills and eye-hand coordination are uninjured, expressing yourself this way helps connect you to the subconscious part of yourself.

Rewards

Every time you practice deep breathing and every time you dip into this book, reward yourself.

What's your favourite reward? A few examples:
- TV show;
- A movie on Netflix;
- Animated movie or series;
- Sitting on a quiet bench in a park;
- Watching squirrels;
- Comfort food, but not too much;
- Chocolate or coffee or tea;
- A walk;
- Gardening.

Choose a reward for each action below, increasing the reward value so that the last action has a unique, high-value reward:
- Deep breathing;
- Reading a page or two or three;
- Starting on an Action Plan;
- Finishing an Action Plan;

- Finishing a Step;
- Finishing the book without doing most of the Action Plans;
- Finishing the book, including doing most of the Action Plans.

For example, I'd watch a short TV show as my reward for five minutes of deep breathing; have a 10 g piece of 70 percent dark chocolate for reading a page; a special coffee drink for starting an Action Plan; a decadent doughnut for finishing an Action Plan; watching a big movie for finishing a Step; and an exquisite dessert from an expensive bakery for finishing the book.

You can tell sweets and chocolate are at the top of my stress-busting favourite reward list! Write your list on a piece of paper and tape it up where it's visible enough to remind you.

A Note on Sweets

The brain uses glucose for fuel. Brain injury demands much more brain fuel than normal, for it needs extra fuel to repair neurons and reconnect neural networks while functioning in an injured state.

Although I recommend following a low-glycemic diet, which is detailed in books available everywhere, for intensive brain work like reading this book, you need to replenish your brain's spent fuel *immediately*. The best way is through something sweet. BUT it can't be a lot else you'll put on weight.

small amounts eaten immediately after cognitive work is the best way to eat treats →

A treat made from whole grain flour is better than from white flour. And preferably, bake or buy cookies, brownies, cakes, etc. made with organic ingredients.

The Freezer Is Your Friend

I keep halved, whole grain cookies, brownies, or chocolate croissants stocked in the freezer. That way, I eat only half a treat, which is what I need, and not have the other half tempt me. Dark chocolate such as 70 percent is an acquired taste but good for your brain and your pain. Avoid candy bars or milk chocolate in the candy aisle.

You can acquire a taste for dark chocolate by building up to it gradually. Begin with 34 percent milk chocolate, then up it to 50, 60, until you reach 70 or 80 percent. Some brands simply taste better than others. Local chocolateries will probably have the best tasting bars in your area; by sticking to 10 g per day as a reward immediately after brain work, you'll reduce the risk of gaining weight while not being so hard on your wallet.

Drinks Without Calories

Black coffee and tea have virtually no calories while providing both taste and energy. If you're used to drinking either or both with milk, cream, non-dairy milks, and/or sugar, the easiest way to get it to black is to reduce the milk and sugar gradually, little by little, over weeks or months. And as you do so, the coffee or tea's innate flavour will become stronger. That's when you switch your brand, if you haven't already, to organic, fair trade. Your immediate thought is probably, *I can't afford that!*

Some thoughts:
- Purchasing coffee and tea this way allows you to try various flavours. Even when brain injury has given a metallic taste to food, you can still discern these flavours when unadulterated. Enjoying different flavours, provides variety to your day and gives you a sense of mastery in the morning.
- Buying organic or fair trade gives you a chance to support small farmers, thus having a positive effect on the planet and our fellow humans. After brain injury, we have so few opportunities to make a difference. This is one way.
- The expense imposes limitations on how much we drink. This is better for our health and our weight. It also turns these drinks into a mindful time. Instead of gulping down without thinking, we enjoy the moment of brewing and consuming at the pace our energy levels allow.
- You can use a special flavour you like—for example, with me, it's organic Darjeeling tea—to reward yourself after a tough Action Plan. A reward with very few calories is rewarding itself!
- One last note: guard against rewards so enticing, you rush reading and working through the Action Plans.

Tolerance. Coffee and tea contain caffeine, which your brain can develop a tolerance to when you drink the same amount at the same time every day. Tolerance occurs when you no longer experience the familiar alertness or pleasant sensation after your rewarding cup of coffee. At that point, you'll naturally increase the amount of coffee or tea in order to feel the reward. That's how the morning cup of coffee increases to two cups then three then...you get the idea. I avoid developing tolerance by varying the time of day when I drink coffee and tea. I also vary the amount. Sometimes, I'll have half a cup; other times a cup or two; and occasionally, I'll have none and choose a non-caffeinated, unsweetened reward drink instead. If you find yourself drinking more than two cups of coffee or tea in a day, gradually pare back the amount and drink it at a slightly different time in order to reduce back down to two or one cup per day. Audiovisual entrainment is a better way to increase your alertness during the day than multiple cups of coffee or tea.

Music and Art

Art in all its forms provides tools with which to grieve and unearth your feelings and thoughts.

Music

Sometimes, simply listening to music that speaks to your loss releases the emotions and thoughts stuck deep inside you. Release your tears, and don't let others put a timetable on you. Grief has its own time. And every person has a unique grief time. Brain injury complicates the grief process because injury itself impairs the ability to grieve. Perhaps you remember how grief felt different, expressed itself differently before your injury? Grieve that change, too, but also tell yourself how you're grieving now is OK.

Art

While music releases emotions, art complements writing in expressing them.
    Use your favourite medium. Paint, crayons, pencils, digital, or collage on paper, parchment, scraps, or tablets.
    My psychologist told me to buy watercolour paints. I went to an art store in downtown Toronto and asked the man behind the counter to help me, for I had no experience with watercolours and needed something easy to use. He didn't judge me but assisted me in gathering paints, brushes, and art paper that suited my beginner level best.
    Find a store like that.

Alternatively, order online and use Amazon reviews to guide you. Even if you don't buy your art supplies from Amazon, their reviews are a good buying guide.

Put your finished pieces where you can see them. Every time you pass that place, rest your eyes on your creations for a bit to continue to help you process. If all your artwork does is make you furious, take the fury-inducing art piece to your therapist and talk it over with them. If you don't have a therapist, perhaps you have a trusted person in your life who can help you, whether online or in person? Or if you have no-one, set up a blog or join social media where you can post your art and write whatever comes out without conscious thought interrupting the process.

Action Plan: Distraction

Distraction is an easy tool to use for escaping trauma pain. It is for me. Distraction gives your brain a break and your heart and mind space.

What distracts you the best?

List Distractions

Open your first notebook *Stress and Grieving*. Title a clean page with "Distractions." Underneath, list your distractions. You may come back to this over time and add to the list or change it as you heal.

Reminder of Top Three Distractions

At the top of a post-it note, write "Distractions" and underline it. Then underneath "Distractions," print your top three distractions. Place the post-it on the cover of your notebook where you'll see your top three list easily and have it remind you.

If your handwriting is unreadable, type out your top three distractions, print out your list, cut it out, and tape it to the cover of your *Stress and Grieving* notebook.

For me, an animated movie on Netflix is one of my top three distractions because animation is funny and easy on my brain. You want something that elicits a smile or a laugh. Even if your injury killed off your laughter, a funny sitcom or movie, especially animation for kids, lightens the load.

CHAPTER 4

PRE-INJURY STRESS BUSTERS

The next step in preparing to heal is to review your stress busters before and after your brain injury. You may have several or one, but let's focus on your core stress busters.

Core Pre-Injury Stress Buster

Before my brain injury, I read loads. A mass paperback book accompanied me everywhere. I read it during lunch, on the subway, in waiting rooms, walking along the street to the disapproval of older adults who thought I'd step onto the road against the red traffic light. Nope. I never did. My amazing brain kept one eye on where I was going and the other engrossed in my novel.

Reading was my stress buster.

My brain injury smashed it into smithereens.

Only one specialist took the grief of losing my reading seriously. Although their clinic understood my pain and tried to help me recover my reading, none seriously believed regaining my pre-injury level of reading was possible. I had to grieve this loss of my core self surrounded by people who either didn't get it or didn't know how to relieve my grief.

Let's Begin

I suspect, like me, you haven't been heard nor given space to grieve your most reliable pre-injury stress buster. And so let's begin by remembering that one and your other pre-injury stress busters. Their loss reduces your stress management tools and increases your stress because you can't access them, you're grieving them deep down in your heart and subconscious, and maybe you don't yet have substitutes that work well for you.

Action Plan: List Your Pre-Injury Stress Busters

Now, let's get to work.

Open your *Stress and Grieving* notebook. Title a fresh page, "Pre-injury Stress Busters." List all your stress busters you used before your injury. Write without thinking.

Now highlight your core one. If you had a couple or three core stress busters, highlight those two or three. Then number them in order of stress-busting power. You're done!

Reward yourself with some down time before moving on to the next Action Plan. Maybe go to the park to soak in Nature or watch a favourite light-hearted TV show.

Action Plan: Grieve Your Pre-Injury Stress Busters

Before we begin, know this may take several sessions to complete because of the emotions and lag time in processing. That's OK. However many sessions it takes or however short those sessions, that's OK. This work is yours; you're doing it to heal yourself. Choose a reward for starting this work, and spend two minutes deep breathing first.

Open your *Stress and Grieving* notebook, and on a new page write, "Core stress buster one." Underneath, copy the top highlighted stress buster from your list.

Then write the story of this stress buster. Begin with its origin and include:
- How did it grow?
- What did it mean to you as a child?
- What did it mean to you as an adult?
- How did it make you feel?
- What did it do for you?
- When did you use it?
- What did other people think of it?
- Did you compromise using it because of adults' or friends' or spousal judgement?
- Do you regret not using it enough?
- What do you miss most about it?

Write a favourite story of using it when it worked well.

Feel the Feelings

Sit for a moment and feel the feelings that come up. Or sit with your thoughts if you have no affect or emotions. Perhaps you have delayed processing and know you won't feel anything for a certain number of hours or days. In that case, schedule a date and time to return to this page when you know the emotions and thoughts will have appeared and your crying and rage will power your writing. Repeat this exercise for your next one or two pre-injury stress busters.

Bringing Abandonment into Consciousness

Reading was my core stress buster. I talked about it to my lawyer, my therapists, my psychologist, my family, my friends, and I wrote on and on about it. For 18 years, I talked, wrote, and sought treatment. The ones who loved me either denied my loss or listened yet offered no practical help. Abandonment stung every cell in my heart.

I wrote about that, too.

Take a moment to write about how loved ones, whom you expected to empathize and perhaps help you, didn't.
- What help did you hope for but didn't receive?
- How did you feel about their abandonment, or what did you think?
- What do you feel or think now about that time?

Perhaps writing has outed your thoughts, but the grief remains. Let's expand your grief's expression with art or music. I'll talk more about grief and healing grief in Steps Three and Four.

Reward

This grieving work is heavy. Reward yourself after each session, whether you spend five minutes or hours on it, whether you complete this entire Action Plan or start but don't finish the story of your top pre-injury stress buster. What will give your brain a break? Make you smile? Help you rest beyond a nap? Do that.

CHAPTER 5

TODAY'S STRESS BUSTERS

Action Plan: Current Stress Busters

Now you've begun grieving your pre-injury stress buster(s), let's list your current stress busters.

Start a new page in your *Stress and Grieving* notebook and title it, "Current Stress Busters."

Write without thinking what they are.

If you're stalled, write what you do when life gets difficult.
- Do you watch TV?
- Load up a movie on Netflix?
- Walk your dog?
- Play with your cat?
- Eat a large chocolate bar?
- Drink more coffee?
- Have a tea ritual?
- Shop online?

- Window shop?
- Sleep?

Now number them in effectiveness.

Which Stress Busters Will You Use?

Highlight in yellow the one(s) you will use after each time you read this book.

Highlight in pink the one(s) you will use after each time you start or follow an Action Plan. This stress buster will be in addition to the reward you've chosen under Tools.

But if you're like me, you'll find that what may've worked early in your brain injury doesn't now, and, as well, your top current ones aren't the healthiest for you. In that case, why not create healthier core ones and ones that come as close as possible to your pre-injury stress busters? Let's start that creative work.

How to Create New Stress Busters

Evolution of One of My Stress Busters

In my teens, I had a spiral-bound Garfield notebook calendar. I think they call that style a desktop calendar these days. It fit in my knapsack and sat on a corner of my desk. I had a ridiculously retentive memory, and I honestly didn't need it. But I loved using coloured pens, chuckling over the cartoons, feeling the tactility of the thick paper.

About a decade later, I was browsing in my favourite pen store and spotted glass pens. A little expensive, but I loved their spiral nibs, the beauty of yellow imprisoned in the clear glass, the idea of writing with ink in the old-fashioned way. I bought it.

Further on in time, I replaced my paper desktop calendar with a FiloFax to plan my wedding then added a Far Side electronic one before software designers made digital calendars all business like.

Then brain injury hit.

A few years into my brain injury life, a homemaker broke my glass pen. I had no affect. And so I shrugged, mentally adding its physical loss to the pile of cognitive losses that included losing my organizational and planning abilities. The person who'd organized herself to the nth degree had become incapable of organizing herself out of a paper bag!

Neurostimulation treatments over the years restored some of this ability, and now and then, I'd have human help. I bought a handheld organizer, the precursor to the Palm and iPhone. But I received no professional help in using it until community care temporarily provided a behavioural therapist who worked with me on my priorities each week. I felt organized and in control. But thinking on my own beyond a week and organizing even one day still feels like a chore that goes nowhere. I tried different paper calendars and hopped from calendar app to calendar app. I tried an ePaper scheduling template and using Google to read out my agenda most mornings. Exasperated doesn't cover how I felt! I needed to create a stress-busting way to organize my day.

But busting stress goes beyond seeing and scheduling priorities.

Professional Advice versus My Changing Brain

To bust my stress, my occupational therapist told me to journal; my psychologist to paint; my church to volunteer. I learnt the key to reducing the stress on a broken brains is going with its ability to work in five-minute increments or to see only an hour into the future or to lift a one-pound or one-kilogram weight or to walk half a block and no more. In the end, I gravitated and stuck with those stress busters that spoke to my core person still in me somewhere, changed yet unchanged.

After losing my pre-injury reading stress buster, and with the frustration of calendar apps that didn't quite work for me, I needed to create new stress busters. The thing about them, like with other aspects of ourselves, is that their effectiveness changes because our brain injury doesn't remain static. Secondary injury and entering an altered life with recovery as our new job, changes how our brain injury manifests and brings in new stressors. As we learn about our new self, we discover things we like that we wouldn't have before the injury, including stress busters. In addition, accelerated healing from neurostimulation or neuromodulation therapies returns lost functions, skills, and talents, changing what works to bust stress.

LEARN MORE

> I detailed in my memoir *Concussion Is Brain Injury: Treating the Neurons and Me* about the experience of secondary injury and sped up healing.
>
> For more on the science of secondary injury, see https://concussionisbraininjury.com/education/what-is-brain-injury/
>
> For neurostimulation therapies, see https://concussionisbraininjury.com/treatments/.

Learn About the Present You

Several years after my brain injury, I sallied out to buy a new skirt to accommodate my chocolate-given girth. As I entered the store, I told myself to consider only what drew me. Forget the old me, the one who liked bold reds and vibrant patterns. I shut down my conscious thoughts and memories and let my feet lead me. As I stood in front of the skirt my feet had led me to, I thought, *I'll never wear this colour. It's so...boring.* Yet the skirt colour felt right; I knew the "boring" thought came out of my memory's depths. I bought the "boring" skirt and loved it.

Similarly, when creating stress busters for who you are today, forget about what you used to like, could do, or did a lot before your brain injury. Let all thoughts and memories go, and let your intuition lead you. Accept where it steers you no matter how much your memory tells you this isn't you. Try it out, see how it feels. If it feels good, write it down in your *Stress and Grieving* notebook and add it to your stress-busting repertoire.

Childhood and Adolescence Give Ideas

Becoming an adult means putting away childish things. Brain injury means getting to revisit them, the fun stuff, the stuff you liked, the activities and ways of doing things that made you smile and lift your heart. The things that released your stress. Maybe it's time to resurrect them!

Starting Is Better than Nothing

A minute or five is better than zero. Pushing yourself to meet others' expectations or trying to be who you were leads to crashing. *Knock it off!* I'd yell at myself. I had to because I was the Queen of pushing myself to crashing and being unable to do anything for a month. Year after year.

Twenty-two years after my injury, I searched Amazon for a desktop calendar with cartoons in it, pages that show at most a week, and spiral bound so that I'm not fighting to keep it open with my limited energy. I wanted one that would give me back the pleasure I used to have in my adolescence, even if I still cannot organize myself well.

As I searched for stickers to go with my new desktop calendar, I stumbled upon glass pens. I bought the most inexpensive one. Bonus: it came with ink colours of varying hues from yellow to pink to purple. I used the same principle I used when I went shopping for that new skirt: I chose the stickers, the calendar, and the glass pen that spoke to me as I am today. Within my budget, of course. That's how I created a new stress buster for taking the stress out of organizing myself. It doesn't work all the time, but it's better than before.

Action Plan: Visual Clutter Stresses

I'll digress here and note what my occupational therapist told me: clutter burdens the injured brain.

Both visual clutter and auditory clutter in the form of noise drains us. I clean and tidy my desk when I can't stand it anymore or when I'm starting a new writing project. And I tidy a small section of my home for 10 minutes in a day, or more when I'm able to or less when I can't. I do what I can when I can. It's better than seeing five minutes as not worth it and so not doing anything.

Once you tidy a place, clutter creeps back in, daring you to put it away. But it's worth the cycling tidying. You'll find your brain goes "Ahhhh" with a cleared desk, leaving just a computer on it and maybe a notebook, desktop calendar, and a charming container for your pens. Or a spot in your living room with a chair and a side table with nothing on it but a lamp and a view to the outdoors (assuming it's not a busy road).

A Quiet Space for This Book

Pick a quiet corner where you'll read this book. Perhaps a chair by a window with a table and lamp beside it. Declutter this space. Have on the table only those tools you need while reading this book. Store them in a drawer or basket at your table's feet. Or if you need their visibility to remind you to read and follow the Action Plans, neaten them on the table so they don't fall off as you dig into your next session.

Every time clutter creeps back in to your quiet space, schedule a moment to declutter it again and reward yourself with a mini but enjoyable treat of your choice when you're done.

Home Devices to Reduce Stress and Anxiety

I have an advantage most people's therapists and doctors haven't given them: home audiovisual entrainment, cranioelectrical stimulation, and photobiomodulation (low-intensity laser) devices. I begin each morning with SMR/Beta brainwave enhancement with my audiovisual entrainment device. It calms my brain and counters the paralyzing effect of my overwhelming life.

Introduced to Audiovisual Entrainment

I first experienced this neurostimulation therapy in my psychologist's office. Most weeks, he'd ask about my week, choose an appropriate audiovisual entrainment protocol, then have me lie back in a zero-gravity chair to relax while the device enhanced the desired brainwave frequencies. I'd feel loads better for a few hours or maybe a couple of days. By my next appointment, I'd be like a person in the Sahara desert coming upon an oasis, hoping the keeper would offer me water. Sometimes my psychologist wouldn't include audiovisual entrainment in our session. Unfortunately, I was incapable of asking for it. I'd leave so disappointed and in despair, I could barely get myself home.

A new psychologist five and a half years after my brain injury referring me to Mind Alive and telling me to purchase a home device, was like being given water in the desert of despair.

audiovisual entrainment counters stress and anxiety →

I recognize most people may not know about neurostimulation therapies like audiovisual entrainment and, as well, their family, physicians, or own fear dissuade them from trying it. I know the inordinate strength required to fight naysayers, to keep at health care professionals until they finally agree to help you, to ignore family and friends who tell you you're being scammed, to fight against the almost crippling anxiety of trying a new therapy, especially on your own and one so unknown to the public and doctors. I know self-advocacy for healing brain injury is arduous and despairing and ends with you feeling like you're defending your right to live. I write about self-advocacy in Step Five.

So I'm writing this book on brain injury, trauma, and grief with the assumption you have no home devices and receive no neurostimulation therapies. But I'm hoping that by the time you finish this book, you'll have the internal healing to go out and fight for the physical healing of your neurons. You're worth it!

LEARN MORE

"It's easier for clients or patients to adopt at-home use of cranioelectrical stimulation when their health care provider introduces them to it during their therapy sessions." https://www.psychologytoday.com/ca/blog/concussion-is-brain-injury/201912/cranioelectrical-stimulation-concussion-and-ptsd

See my *Psychology Today* blog at https://www.psychologytoday.com/ca/blog/concussion-is-brain-injury for more.

For the neuroscience behind these medical technologies, see https://concussionisbraininjury.com/treatments/.

I wrote about my experience in my memoir *Concussion Is Brain Injury: Treating the Neurons and Me*.

Action Plan: Create New Stress Busters

Let's create new core stress busters to add to your current repertoire. They may be a combination of returning pre-injury ones plus new ones that suit the new you.

Childhood and adolescence were when we got to do things that were playful. Living with brain injury is a long road of pain. We need stress busters that incorporate fun and are doable within our limited energy and strength.

Think fun! →

On a fresh page of your *Stress and Grieving* notebook, write at the top, "Create New Stress Buster."

Whimsy

What whimsical thing did you do as a child or teen that you remember with fondness? That, in this moment, the memory lifts your spirit?

I'm not talking about something you did with others, but something you did for yourself and by yourself or something you desired but had no chance to try.

List everything that comes to mind.

A Good Thing You Gave Yourself

What did you give yourself as a young adult when you embarked on your working life?

As you wander through your memory banks, search for something small, preferably inexpensive, that gave you pleasure.

List everything that comes to mind.

Review Your Two Lists

Now review your lists and check off the ideas that are doable now as stress busters, given your energy, current abilities, and budget limitations.

Consider, too, modifying one or combining two into one doable stress buster. For example, I combined my cartoon desktop calendar from my high school years with the glass pen from my early adulthood. When I write in my calendar, I choose an ink colour that matches the week's colour. Sometimes, I'll use my glass pen to write my ToDos for the day or that week's goal; other times I'll use a marker or my fountain pen. Add your combined stress-buster idea to one of your lists and check it off.

How does it make you feel reading these new stress busters in black and white on the page?

Number each item in your list in order of preference and feasibility and start testing them.

Try your top one first for a month. As you use it, do you find it busts your stress a little bit or a lot? Are you using it less and gravitating back to your less healthy stress busters as the month wears on? You'll find that you're more likely to stick with the new stress buster if it's fun and resonates with your core self. Yes, brain injury means you forget, you tire, you find you haven't used it for a week or more. But that's OK, that's the nature of brain injury. You'll return to using it if it works and when you remember. Test your next listed new stress busters in the following months until you've created a list of three healthy, effective stress busters you'll use reliably. These top three may be just your newly created ones or ones you had developed before reading this book or a combination of both.

Disappearing Habits

Soon after my car crash, my physiotherapist gave me a regimen of light weights to do three times a week. She probably wanted me to lift weights more often for the sake of my bones and strengthening my sprained muscles, but that's all the energy I had. Weights, when properly sized to current strength and energy capabilities, reduce pain and give energy. I scheduled them in my calendar app. What I didn't know is that when exercise frequency and time extend beyond the brain's capacity to regulate the heart, energy turns into shortness of breath and water retention that puffs the face. I struggled with both for years as I strained to exercise normally. After all, exercise benefits the brain! The experts neglect to consider how exercise affects the injured brain.

Almost a decade after my crash, a physical trainer who worked with concussed elite athletes taught me my shortness of breath and puffy face came from too much exercise. He reduced my weight training to ten minutes three times a week. "Weight training" makes it sound like I'm lifting dumbbells at a gym. Nope, little one-pounders in my home.

Since the weights made me feel better and I'd formed a better exercise habit, I figured I didn't need to schedule them anymore. Bad idea. Habits don't stick in an injured brain. Memory doesn't work like that in us. I completely forgot to do them for two weeks. I put weights and walking back in my calendar.

Scheduling Overcomes Habit Loss

list your top three stress busters and pin them in a visible location on a wall or fridge

So whatever your stress busters are, from regular five-minute walks to watching a movie to watching passersby on the street, write them down to remind you. Schedule the exercise ones. Put your journal right next to your bed where its visibility reminds you to write in it. Place your food rewards such as chocolate in a cupboard out of sight so that you don't gorge on them, but when you open the cupboard door, the sight of good-quality 70 percent dark chocolate reminds you 10 g of chocolate is your reward for completing an Action Plan or reading a chapter.

CHAPTER 6

TIME

What Do You Want?

Before you dig into Step One, write what you want on a card.
What talents, skills, abilities, social life, work, vacations, way of being do you want?

Distill this list into a simple statement or image. For example, "I want to heal my trauma and neurons for a better life."

I assume you picked up this book and want to work through it because your desire includes having your brain injury fully healed. A full cure of injury and trauma may not be possible, but it is possible to heal wounds and to heal neurons with neurostimulation and neuromodulation treatments based on the right diagnostics. First, though, you need the wherewithal to fight for it. Gaining that begins with processing your brain injury grief, learning that deep down you're loved, and coming to believe you're worth being restored.

Now that you've written your goal on a card, sign and date it. Then pin the card somewhere prominent where it'll catch your attention as you go about your day. Tell yourself when you see it, "This is worth working towards."

Time

Time stalks us like a hungry lion, commanding all our attention. We hear it creeping behind us, ahead of us, pulling us in its direction, not ours.

Tick. Tick. Tick. I heard the steady movement of the clock, counting out days, weeks, months, then years of time lost to my brain injury. A day without treatment meant a day lost to me.

"You're late!" came the inevitable complaint from myself and others because no matter how hard I tried, time slipped away from me, and I'd arrive at my destination behind time.

Time Persuades Us to Judge

Our collective sense of time, the necessity of meeting health care providers at their stated time, leads to us being seen as failing to heed others' needs...except in some clinics that believe in creating a stress-free environment. For them, time doesn't matter; treating the patients matters.

Those who've read my memoir *Concussion Is Brain Injury: Treating the Neurons and Me* will have seen the deleterious effect of time ruling my mind, of rushing and pushing myself back towards normal.

Einstein revealed the relativity of time to us over a century ago. We understand that as we speed faster and faster, time slows down. We also, sort of, understand time-space changed over the centuries so that if we go back in time, we also have to shift in space in order to land in the same space as we currently inhabit.

But what about internal time?

An Injured Brain's Internal Clock

It's said time is slower for children than adults, and elderly people experience time as speeding faster and faster. After my brain injury, time slowed to a crawl. I re-experienced childhood time. An hour became a day. A day like a week. Yet something else happened, too. My processing speed plummeted to the basement. I both perceived time as slower externally and time as normal internally.

Let me try to explain.

Automaticity Affects Time Perception

Automaticity is when you do or sense something automatically without conscious thought or effort. Automaticity takes less brain power and is faster than conscious thought. Prior to brain injury, you brushed your teeth and didn't remember doing it because your brain had learned to do that automatically from years of practice, starting in childhood. As an adult, you no longer need to attend to each stroke of your toothbrush to know you've brushed your teeth. You've achieved automaticity. That freed up your mind to think about other things, and the act of brushing your teeth whipped by. After brain injury destroyed automaticity, you had to again consciously think through every action in brushing your teeth in order to complete it. Now brushing your teeth feels like an hour.

My perception of action that had lost its automaticity, whether brushing my teeth or making breakfast or catching a bus, stretched their time consumption. How did a half hour pass by for something that takes me five minutes? So puzzling! Now I know: doing something with conscious thought takes much longer than after developing automaticity.

In addition, the act of consciousness meant I was aware of every second of the effort. Time felt longer. Since the car crash had damaged my sensory perception, too, every act of sensory input became conscious instead of automatic.

And another strangeness: We with brain injury lose time. We may look out the window for a couple of minutes then turn to look at the clock and see 30 minutes have passed. What is happening in our brain that we lose time in this way?

Internal Perception versus Perception of Me by Others

Every time I met with my yoga instructor back in 2007, my internal perception of time mismatched external time. I'd be doing ten reps of an exercise, and she'd be telling me to speed up, and I'd be thinking, *I'm zooming along, what's she talking about?!* So puzzling! And aggravating for both of us!!

I believe what was happening relates to my slower-than-frozen-molasses processing speed.

As healthy people, our internal perception of how quick we are—that is, movement in time—dovetails with others' perception. I theorize we have this internal sense of time connected to our collective sense of time because our brains share relatively the same processing speed. Speech reflects this concept well.

I met with a newish friend for coffee and told her about my brain injury. Understanding lit her eyes and relaxed her face. She said, "I thought something was wrong. Your speech doesn't match your intelligence. My brothers are intelligent, and they speak faster than you. You should be speaking like them."

speech reflects processing speed →

Those with much quicker processing speeds will be seen as speaking quickly all the time; the opposite for those with much slower.

Yet, no matter our outward speed, I believe our internal perception of our own thinking, feeling, and acting feels like normal time. And that normal time dovetails relatively well with the collective sense of normal time.

Except for the outliers, either highly intelligent or delayed, most tick along with enough similarity that we don't feel that far apart in our sense of normal speed.

But brain injury throws us out of that collective sense. It makes our perception of moving in normal time—our speed—completely different from most people's. As a result, the yoga instructor, from her outward perception, saw my movements as slow, while I saw them, from my inward perception, as speedy.

That also means that an act we know from before our injury takes a minute, like putting on socks, ends up after brain injury feeling like it stills takes a minute but in actuality takes much longer. We feel internally that we're putting our socks on in normal time, like we did before brain injury, yet when we look at the clock, it relentlessly informs us that five minutes have passed. That confusing disconnect takes years to accommodate to when no one acknowledges or explains it to us.

Bottom Line?

We have two problems with time. Every action requiring conscious effort means both taking longer and feeling endless. And just as time is relative in the universe, it's also relative internally. Injury destroys our internal connection to the external in two ways.

- Whatever our processing speed is, we perceive it internally as normal time.

- Brain-injured processing speed disconnects our sense of normal time from the collective sense of normal time.

These two changes lead to us losing time, feeling like we're rushing yet being late, and being seen as super slow when we feel normal inside.

neurostimulation treatments restore automaticity and re-sync our normal time to the collective normal time

Until then, we have to readjust our schedules to accommodate that conscious effort and our injured internal clock.

Bottom Bottom Line?

Forget about time when healing. Treatments and returning to health takes as long as it takes.

Releasing myself from the confining demands of time allowed me to keep at my reading practice when it was a dispiriting five minutes a day for months. Turning my back on the passing years allowed me to go back to those things that gave me pleasure in my childhood, adolescence, and early adulthood: the Garfield calendar, the colourful pens, the glass pen, and fun ink colours.

Releasing yourself from time will allow you to read this book and heal from brain injury in the way your mind and neurons can handle. Your life has a purpose, and time cannot stop it, even when it feels like we've lost decades to this catastrophic injury. To those who want you to be chained to the collective sense of time, give a silent raspberry while outwardly giving them a copy of this section.

Recap: Preparing to Read This Book

To recap Step Zero: Preparation. Before, during, and after each time you pick up this book, do the following.
1. Remind yourself of your goal.
2. Deep breathe for two minutes.
3. Ready your stress buster(s) to use during and after reading this book and following the Action Plans.

4. If you haven't decided on a reward yet for your current reading session, choose one. Something small that will make you feel good. I have dark chocolate because brain work requires glucose and dark chocolate provides the fuel my brain needs to replenish itself and makes my taste buds happy.
5. Gather your notebook, pens, stickers, and whatever other fun tools you have to follow the Action Plans.
6. Sit in your quiet space free of visual and auditory clutter.
7. Even though I'll talk later about energy conservation, pacing during a cognitively demanding task can help—except if you forget where you were and have to restart every time you take a break. In that case, build in extensive rest time afterwards.
8. Set a timer for however long you can read before neuro-fatigue sets in. That may only be five minutes or ten at a time, and that's OK. When the timer goes off, stand up and stretch.
9. Remind yourself time doesn't matter. It's reading for understanding and doing the work that matters. Release yourself from the calendar's and others' urgency and notice how you feel better when you don't rush but give each section the time it and you deserve.
10. Ask yourself out loud at the end of each section or paragraph:
    A. Summarize what you read.
    B. What does this make me think of?
    C. What can I conclude?
    D. What does this mean to me?
    E. Do I agree or disagree with Shireen and why?
11. Reread or redo whatever you have to.
12. Reward yourself immediately. Even clapping to yourself, pumping your arms in the air, putting a smile on your face, are rewards for a job well done! You put in the effort. Now time to celebrate!
13. Use your stress buster to cool down.

HEALING
Begins
With
KNOWING
You're **LOVED**
And with
Grieving *your lost life*

Step One

LOVED AND UNLOVED

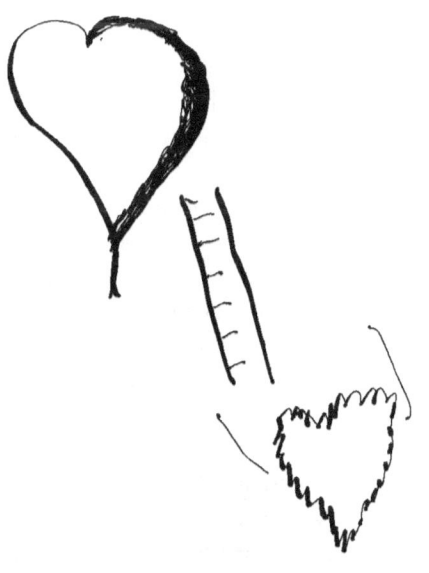

CHAPTER 7

A NEW WORD: MITHRA!

Before healing can begin, we need to know who we are, really are. We are not what we do; not what others judge; not static beings. We're a beloved creation.

> "All of a sudden, I felt Jesus near me as if he was a golden light around and speaking within me. I knew without a doubt that Jesus loved me. It didn't matter that I was considered a brat, bossy, stubborn, relentlessly asking questions, too dark, light, too small. Jesus loved the whole of me. And then the presence was gone. It was back to normal in that room except that my heart sang that at least one being loved me no matter what."
>
> *From* Concussion Is Brain Injury: Treating the Neurons and Me, Chapter 1: Y2K.

I used the word "loved" because that's the word I know. English has hundreds of thousands of words and only one word for every kind of love. One word, so many meanings. Yet the word "love" is inadequate to what I experienced. I had no clue who Jesus was. Adults and children my age (six years old) knew, but I couldn't understand who this person was that they kept talking about. Then, in that moment, I felt the presence of a big brother, a friend, exterior to me, and part of me, loving me in almost every kind of way and creating love in me.

Over the years, I've thought about our social biology and how a glue binds us human beings together so that individuals thrive and the species survives. That glue is another kind of love. Yet, again, the word "love" is inadequate. We need a new word to describe this specific glue. *Mithra*.

Mithra Definition

Mithra—that which interconnects all humans to every human through space-time, is both a biological contract and a thinking-emotion, and is the foundation which holds up every kind of love.

Mithra ripples outward as we influence others, near and far. And mithra ripples inward as both those we know and those we don't know influence us. No one is an island, even when loved ones, society, and governments try to strand us on one. This is why I can't stand the phrase, "God doesn't give us more than we can handle." Of course, God does! This blaming-the-victim phrase infers God expects us to be able to stand alone and succeed alone—or with only God supporting us.

God gave us each other to help us through the tough times →

When done without expectation of payback and out of a giving heart, supporting each other intrinsically rewards and strengthens every party—helper, helpee, and beyond. Nature built mithra expression into our genes.

> "If one person had a problem, everyone intervened to help. This selflessness made it evident…how much they prioritized each other's needs over their own comfort.
>
> Much of our time on Earth is spent undoing the barriers that prevent us from giving and receiving love. Fear, doubt, and apathy keep us stuck."
>
> *From Tyler Henry*, Here & Hereafter, *observing and describing mithra.*

Dr. Bruce Perry related his visit with a Maori community in *What Happened To You?* He learnt that "reciprocal relationships, kinship, and a sense of family connection" were integral to their healing practices. The family connection extended far beyond the nuclear family. Family, in this sense, encompassed what we from India call Aunty and Uncle—any adult who comes into our lives and forms a connection with us. Healing in this community involved reconnecting, either symbolically or literally, outward from family to community to Nature. And Nature, community, and family came together to heal their sick member. Their healing practice honours mithra.

Unfortunately, people whose loved one has a brain injury spend their time putting up barriers to exclude the injured one out of fear, and we, the injured, spend years trying to futilely break through those barriers. Many ignore mithra and focus only on love of "acceptable" members within a family or close friendships, while romantic love is the one most sung and written about. But without mithra, there is no romantic, family, sisterly, brotherly, neighbourly, or friendship love. Mithra undergirds all.

What Kind of Love Do We Need?

Since the time of Old English in the 700s, love's meaning has changed from the idea of love between God and human to today's idea of a sexual relationship between two people, or the lesser idea of love between family members or best friends. Each of these concepts excludes all others outside of the couple, family, or group. It's no wonder our societies have devolved into "every man is his own castle." Which, by the way, is false. No one person can succeed alone. People who mount fortresses between themselves and others grow loneliness, for we were built to work together. Our brains measure closeness and map people in our social space. We are social beings, and mithra is the glue that binds us together across space-time. Mithra is what allows us to thrive as individuals and to survive as a species.

you were loved into being

The Creation story of God bringing the world into being is all about love: of God for humans and mithra between humans. Love and mithra create and maintain relationships. A creator imagines characters into existence, fills them with life, revels in telling their stories, relates to them, and never wants to let them go, including the "bad ones." So God, being a creator, loved us into being.

Sir Roger Penrose, the Nobel-winning mathematrical physicist, doesn't believe in God, yet believes in a conscious cosmos. He marvels at how atoms came together to create you and me!

you exist in mithra →

And so what a travesty that we exist alone, isolated because of our brain injury and the castle mentality of our world, where society confines steadfast love to two people who have sex.

Yes, we use the word "love" for family members. But we're judged, rejected, and abandoned because humans ignore mithra and so can judge us as no longer meeting the conditions for family or friendship love. Or being suitable for a productive society. Or even exist.

What a travesty that love, whether God's unconditional creation or Nature's amazing randomness, has devolved into this one-dimensional idea of love that holds only under human-imposed conditions and denies the existence of mithra.

A Note to You, Valued Reader

God and Nature: My Approach

I'll digress here to note that I come from a Zoroastrian and Christian background. Both religions have informed my life. Yet weirdly, I've rarely had Christian friends and no Zoroastrian friends, though I've socialized with both. One of my earliest friends in Canada is an atheist, and I empathize with why they don't believe in God. Sometimes, I wonder why I do! Not because of the usual reasons people put forth, but because the relationship is so painful.

Yet these last 22 years would've been impossible for me to survive without that relationship. It matters that when no one loves you, you know that Jesus or God absolutely does. I think it's time I stopped being shy about my philosophy, my relationship with Jesus and God—and about mithra.

Before my encounter with Jesus at six years old, I didn't understand who this person was that all the other children knew. In that encounter, I instantly did. Since then, I've spent most of my life studying, discussing, thinking about God, Jesus, the Creation stories from both religions, the central themes of each, as well as theoretical physics, psychology, and neurophysiology. My brain injury opened up the challenging vista of philosophy of mind. My Pastor enjoyed the heretical nature of my faith and discussing the concepts behind my novels. When I was preparing to write *Lifeliner* before my brain injury, I learnt about the four pillars that allow people to not just survive a catastrophic illness, but also thrive.

Relationships and faith are two of the four key pillars. These both revolve around love and rest on the foundation of mithra. (The other two are the relationship with your medical team and their competence, and having a strong will and goal.)

Drawing From Learnings

After my brain injury, I studied the *Book of Job* with my Pastor, co-lead a group bible study on it, then wrote an ebook with handouts. I draw from that ebook in this book. But I also draw from my experiences and learnings in the last 22 years after my brain injury. Today, we're realizing that, like peoples in ancient times, you don't need an MD or Ph.D. to be an expert. Experience and willingness to learn the unfamiliar are what good experts do. The only difference is whether or not an institution gives you a credential for such.

Whenever I mention God in this book, I use the neutral pronoun "they" as simultaneously singular and plural. When you study the original vocabulary, the pronouns are female, male, and neutral. Since we are all made in the image of God, it's logical God exists beyond gender yet encompasses every gender form.

When I mention God, I'll give the Nature perspective, too, for I know that whether or not you believe God exists, everyone with a brain injury is hurting. And everyone deserves to have their beliefs respected and spoken to. We exist, after all, in mithra.

CHAPTER 8

GOD OR NATURE

God

When I write novels, I like to think about the characters, work out their stories, write the ending before the beginning so that I know no matter how tortuous their paths, my main character ends up in the place I want them to. God is a storyteller at the cosmos level, their Creation beyond comprehension for its complexity and numbers of characters—us—weaving our paths independently and together.

God created you and me—loved us into being—out of who they are.

God exists beyond us and within us. It's rather mind blowing to conceive of a being that can see us, hear us, relate to us as individuals while simultaneously existing outside the universe. For like a writer exists outside of their story while inhabiting it, so too does God with their Creation. God doesn't want to let us go, always sees us as their beloved children. God created a planet to nourish our life, with all the elements we need to thrive together, united to each other through mithra, to live in unity with God.

Unity and Mithra

Unity doesn't mean conformity or agreement without thought. Unity means that we each have a role to play within a harmonious whole. Like mithra creates the foundation for every kind of love to flourish, we each have unique skills and talents; personalities and perspectives, that create a whole greater than any individual. Our social biology works best in unity. Our brains connect in person but also across distances, in virtual spaces, down phone lines, across time. Brains support brains, explained one of my clinicians when I found reading easier when seated next to another human being. Our brains connect to keep, grow, support and be supported in relationships. That's how God created us.

Nature

Theoretical physics posits the Big Bang. But the mathematical physicist Sir Roger Penrose theorized the universe didn't begin with a bang but as a Big Bounce. The universe expanded until it collapsed upon itself. It became so compressed that it exploded out again as a reactive force to the compression. We call that explosive reaction "the Big Bang." The universe is expanding today; eventually, said Penrose, it'll contract again into an infinitesimal space. He called the cycling of expansion and contraction "the Big Bounce."

At the moment, our universe is expanding. At some point, it will begin to collapse, re-entering the cycle of collapsing, exploding, expanding again, and so on. I'm setting aside theories about the multiverse for the purposes of this book.

Whether Big Bang or Big Bounce, our universe came into being billions of years ago. Mystery shrouds its earliest moment, the Planck epoch. Photons and electrons came blazing out of that mystery. And billions of years later, light and energy coalesced into you. What a wondrous happening that a universe so expansive, so enormous that we cannot comprehend it, even when looking up at the stars and galaxies beyond our Milky Way, created you. There's a mithra in that randomness. You are part of the universe; the universe's essential elements are in you, as is true of every single human being. Mithra, the glue that binds us to each other biologically, arose out of what created us.

Why Alone?

So why are we alone when, whether we believe in God or no God, we're meant to live in relationships resting on the foundation of mithra?

I think this is what the words in the Christian prayer "we have erred and strayed like lost sheep" mean—we are easily led away from mithra, away from our hurt loved ones who need our support and encouragement. Or we forget that the Zoroastrian core belief of good thoughts, good words, good deeds entails resisting bad thoughts—for bad thoughts lead to bad words and rationalizing bad deeds, such as isolating a person with brain injury instead of rallying around them.

We forget God sees us all as their children. Or we don't think about how we were all created out of those first photons and electrons of the universe. We forget we thrive because of mithra—that which interconnects us across space-time—and we're only just learning that our brains map a closeness dimension for people we meet in our social space. Our brains are wired to keep people close and to know where we are relative to them. The closeness dimension helps us predict who will be there for us. Unfortunately, it seems that brain injury derails our predictions. Those with the closest of close dimensions too often are not there for us. They oppose their nature when they abandon us with brain injury out of fear. Forgetting and ignoring mithra gives people licence to divide themselves from those who make them uncomfortable—to unlove a loved one.

Action Plan: Contemplate Being Loved

Ponder one or both of these ideas:
1. How God so loved you they imagined you, created you, placed you here in this time and space and doesn't want to ever let you go.
2. The universe created you in this space-time and exists within you and holds you within its vastness because you're an essential part of it.

Sit for a moment in your quiet space with the idea that best fits your beliefs of how you were created. Or go outside and lean against a tree. Or if there's no tree near you or you don't have the energy to move, sit near one of your houseplants or find a photo of a beautiful tree in full bloom to look upon. Rest your eyes on Nature for a moment.

Now write on a piece of paper, "You are in God's care." Or "The universe created and wants you." Look for a picture of a hand cradling a child, like God or the universe is cradling you. Pin or tape the verse and image side by side to your wall near your computer or next to the bathroom mirror, somewhere where you will see them daily. Even when you no longer see them consciously because of familiarity, your brain will still register the message at some level. Like with me, when my mentors recommended doing this, I hope these reminders will nudge a bit of hope into you when it gets too much. You are not your injury, you are part of mithra, and you're loved, no matter what anyone says!

CHAPTER 9

WHAT IS RELATIONSHIP?

Closesness Is a Dimension

Mary-Frances O'Connor writes in *The Grieving Brain* that our brain creates maps of ourself and others in the posterior cingulate cortex. These maps physically represent ourself and people in our lives. Even after they die, loved ones remain physically present in our brains. Kind of remarkable!

Brain Maps

The posterior cingulate cortex is part of the limbic lobe, a deep brain structure that is involved in our emotional responses, memory, and other functions, which researchers continue to learn about. This cortex also encodes where a person is in our social space and their closeness dimension. I wrote on our brain maps of self in the chapter Relationship With Ourself.

We know about space and time dimensions, but did you know closeness is a dimension? The right inferior parietal lobule measures distance and relative distances of objects or people in space, time, and *closeness*. It's strange to think about how the brain can measure closeness and encodes that measurement, but it does. The closeness dimension is part of mithra—it tells us who's important in our lives, who we're important to, and where they are in our social space.

In 1992, psychologist Arthur Aron devised an Inclusion of Other in the Self scale. Looking at a pictogram of circles that represent increasing inclusion of another in their sense of self, a person points to the set that best represents a particular relationship. It, in essence, measures our closeness dimension..

Self's Closeness Dimensions with Others

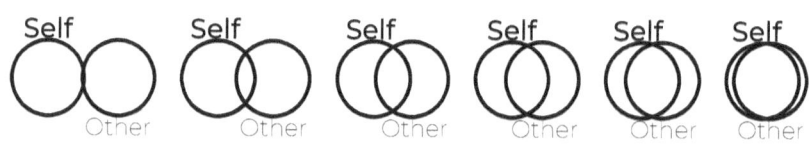

When a person dies, they remain mapped in our brain. Our brain tries to marry the person being gone with its internal physical map and related closeness dimension and biases towards the map over the external reality. We know they're dead, but our brain's hardwired encoding of their existence creates the belief that they will return. To reconcile the existing brain map and closeness dimension with external reality, our brain decides we haven't made enough of an effort to reach out to that person. It creates regret, guilt, and/or anger, social emotions that motivate us to go to the other person and bring them back so that external reality matches our brain's physical mapping once again.

Damage

"It was because your loved one lived, and because you loved each other, that means when the person is no longer in the outer world, they still physically exist—in the wiring of the neurons of your brain."

From The Grieving Brain, *Chapter 3.*

Funerals, condolences, seeing our loved one's dead body serves to provide the physical proof needed to rewire the posterior cingulate cortex's brain maps, thus re-synchronizing the belief with the knowing. Avoiding these actions or rituals delays re-synchronizing.

What happens when brain injury damages the map of your loved one who is still alive? What happens when brain injury erases their closeness dimension and location in your social space? It would be like erasing their existence from your brain, the belief they exist.

I think this may explain why, when anyone we know is out of our sight, they are out of our mind as if they don't exist.

But when they return and show themselves physically existent, it tells our brain they exist. How long they interact with us, how much they help and comfort us, determines if neurons will fire in a particular pattern, encoding a permanent map in our posterior cingulate cortex. But damage to the posterior cingulate cortex and/or right inferior parietal lobule could impede creating brain maps of new people, prevent encoding their closeness dimension, and mapping where they exist in our social space. Then when the loved one leaves, they no longer physically exist either in front of us or perhaps in our brain's hardwiring. As you can imagine, that would make forming new relationships difficult.

Since brain injury can damage one function but not another, we may retain brain maps of persons we knew in our lives prior to brain injury, only bits and pieces of those maps, or none at all. Even if previous brain maps remain, we may lose to injury their related closeness dimension and social space encoding. That could lead to knowing loved ones exist while losing a sense of closeness and certainty where they are in our social space.

Damaged working, short-term, and facial recognition memory could also affect this encoding. As a result, we may neither believe a person is close nor remember they exist. And so, in a subconscious effort to keep them in our mind, we may develop a repetitive need to know where each loved one, or important-to-us person, is at all times. We may feel this need most acutely for those we depend on, such as mothers and health care professionals, and people we're trying to hang on to, such as siblings and best friends.

Another Reason to Receive Neurostimulation

Gradually, over the years, my brain has regained the belief, the knowing that people in my life continue to exist when they're out of sight. It remains difficult for me to feel a connection not only because of brain damage to these areas but also because of traumatic changes in our relationships. Even so, neurostimulation treatment returned to me the ability to have important-to-me people continue to exist in my mind when I haven't seen them for a day or a week or a year.

As neurostimulation heals the posterior cingulate cortex, right inferior parietal lobule, and related structures, and restores memory, our brains will once again be able to encode changes or additions to maps of ourself and others, to closeness dimensions, and to where others exist in our social space. We will no longer feel like we're in a sea of not knowing, not believing, and not remembering that loved ones exist. We won't have to keep asking, checking, searching for where a therapist is or our mother is or our best friend will be to counter out of sight, out of mind. Our brains will know.

Transactional versus Attachment Bonds

In psychology, there are two types of bonds involved in the closeness dimension. Transactional and attachment.

Transactional Bonds

Transactional bonds involve an accounting of who does what, when, where, and how much. A transactional bond tracks how much effort and time each has put into a relationship or teamwork to ensure it's equal, such as with colleagues. When we resent putting in more time and effort into a relationship than the other person, that's a transactional bond. When someone accuses us of demanding too much of their time, that's a transactional bond.

Attachment Bonds

We usually find attachment bonds between close friends and family. They're defined by:
1. We help each other when needed.
2. We spend time together.
3. The person is special, distinct in our brain from other people in our life.

Attachment bonds include empathy. Psychologists define empathy as comprising three aspects:
1. **Cognitive perspective taking**. We're able to see the other person's perspective. For example, we perceive they feel fear at catching brain injury when they look at how tough ours is on us.
2. **Emotional empathy**. We feel what the other person is feeling. For example, when the other person feels sad, we catch their sadness and feel sad, too, in harmony with them.
3. **Compassion**. After we experience cognitive perspective taking and emotional empathy, we feel motivated to help, comfort, or care for the other's well-being. Compassion is empathy in action.

Was It an Attachment Bond?

One of the hardest things about experiencing relationship changes after brain injury is discovering that what we thought was an attachment bond was actually a transactional bond. People drift away from us—or label us—in a way that reflects their resentment over giving to us more than we can give to them. They treat us as a person who vacuums up all their time and doesn't give back to them or the relationship. Attachment bonds don't care about that sort of thing.

Despair fills our heart when we know we can never provide equal effort, time, and skill to a transactional relationship. Our neuro-fatigue, stamina, damaged skills and talents, and so on, limit how much we can do; as a result, we require a lot of support, encouragement, and caring for. We depend on attachment bonds, people in our life who will roll with our brain injury limitations and help us out without resentment or fear.

Action Plan: List Relationship Types

This is a quick Action Plan. It's to help you discern the bonds you had before your brain injury.

Take your *Relationships* notebook out. Title a fresh page, "Bonds." Underneath on the left side of the page, list all the people in your life from before your brain injury, one name per line.

Now reflect on each person you've listed. What did your brain injury reveal about their bond with you? To the right of each name, write your answer: "transactional" or "attachment." Write a question mark if you can't decide. Maybe take this list to your therapist, if you have a health care professional to talk to, or clergy, and go over it with them, especially the ones you can't figure out if they were transactional when you'd thought they were attachment.

Reward yourself when done.

Faces

When we meet someone, our fusiform gyrus records their face, which allows us to recognize that person in new situations and different circumstances. Because of this ability, we can meet our occupational therapist in the clinic and recognize them on the street; we can strike up a friendship in the waiting room and recognize the new friend when we meet up for coffee the next day; we meet a cousin as teenagers and recognize them years later on a visit across the pond.

Brain injury can kibosh that ability.

Since brain injury can damage one area but leave others intact, we may end up with an inability to recognize familiar faces yet know who someone is. Or we may recognize the face of our occupational therapist but not remember what they do or where they're located in our social space. Or we may not remember their face or who they are, while still recognizing their name. The latter situation causes confusion, uneasiness, distress, despair at knowing a name but not the person. We desire escape because it's so unnerving and alienating.

How do you tell someone you don't know who they are?

You've probably seen these situations distress a friend or family member who refuses to learn about brain injury. Even those who read up on brain injury or have seen your qEEG, evoke potentials, or SPECT scan reports, can still believe subconsciously you don't care about them.

We're not wired to respond well to being forgotten and unknown.

People who want to maintain attachment bonds to us must work with a therapist to find ways to stay connected with us and grieve the loss of being known. Helping you access neurostimulation treatments will ease their grief, too, as it heals these areas.

Mirror Neurons and Oxytocin

Neurons are minuscule cells in our brains that talk to each other via chemical signals called "neurotransmitters" and electrical conductance along their bodies, the axons. Different types do different things. Wired together, firing together, they create neural networks. Electroencephalography uses electrodes pasted to our scalp to pick up our neural networks' electrical activity, called "brainwaves," and measures both the brainwaves' power and frequencies.

Electroencephalography or EEG was first used on humans almost a century ago. Although we know a lot about neurons, we remain on the edge of discovery. Recently, researchers discovered mirror neurons in humans. Mirror neurons do what the name implies: they mirror what we see or hear.

Mirror Neurons

> A type of sensory-motor cell, the mirror neuron activates "when an individual performs an action or observes another individual performing the same action. Thus, the neurons 'mirror' others' actions. Mirror neurons are of interest in the study of certain social behaviours, such as empathy and imitation, and may provide a mechanistic explanation for social cognition."
> *From* Encyclopedia Britannica.

Mirror neurons are involved in imitation and in understanding intention, that is, predicting what an observed person will do next. What's fascinating is that mirror neurons seem to be behind the "Theory of Mind." They allow our brain to construct a model of the thoughts and intentions of the person we're observing or listening to—the ability to predict and make sense of other people's behaviour. They mirror others' thoughts in ourselves.

mirror neurons also mirror emotions.
⎯⎯⎯⎯⎯⎯⎯⎯⎯⎯⎯➤

The Theory of Mind "states that children use their own emotions to predict what others will do. Therefore, we project our own mental states onto others. Mirror neurons are activated both when actions are executed, and the actions are observed. This unique function of mirror neurons may explain how people recognize and understand the states of others; mirroring observed action in the brain as if they conducted the observed action."

From Mirror neurons: Enigma of the metaphysical modular brain.

Modelling is a type of learning that imitates what we see adults doing. Human beings model each other as a form of unconscious learning. When we're with an angry person, we model their way of interacting with customer service, with shouts and threats. But if we're with a calm person who we see and hear speaking politely and kindly to customer service, we'll model that behaviour both at the time and later when we're on our own.

Oxytocin

You've probably heard of oxytocin as the love hormone, the chemical our bodies secrete in a romantic relationship. Seeing love as solely romantic or sexual biases research and reporting on oxytocin studies. Far more exciting to talk about a hormone involved in sex than in friendship, never mind mithra, which interconnects human beings to help individuals, societies, and our species thrive.

Oxytocin floods areas of the brain that also have receptors for serotonin and dopamine, the two neurotransmitters involved in many aspects of brain function including healthy mood.

Nucleus accumbens. The nucleus accumbens rewards us when we do something good for our health and survival. When we're with someone who treats us well—who looks and sounds like they want to be with us—oxytocin streams out of our neurons in the nucleus accumbens. This flood, when we're in the presence of another person who's spending time with us, helping us, and standing out from the crowd, permits the brain to strengthen our attachment bond with that person. Having strong attachment bonds is rewarding. It not only feels good to be attached, talking, laughing, hanging out, it also means that when we're in trouble, we'll have help and vice versa. Human beings working together survive better and longer than individuals working alone. Yes, being alone is bad for our health, but that doesn't mean we give up!

Friendship Has Health Consequences

When loved ones declare us toxic and socially isolate us, they in fact create a toxic outpouring of the stress hormone cortisol in both us and in themselves. But whereas they can calm this stress reaction by forming new relationships, our social isolation coupled with our brain-injured inability to form bonds means we cannot. We remain in a permanent state of cortisol activation. (I described it in my memoir *Concussion Is Brain Injury: Treating the Neurons and Me* as looking like the Michelin Man. Too much cortisol from many stressors over time leads to one looking like they're on steroids.)

Researchers have delved into explaining friendship scientifically by studying its underlying mechanisms, development, evolutionary origins, biological function, and neural networks. They call this "neuroethology" and suggest that understanding it helps us understand the essential bonds of friendship and what disrupts them. Disrupted social bonds lead to health problems, shorter lifespans, and difficulties forming or maintaining friendships.

I would argue the other way around also happens in brain injury. Injury to mirror neurons, to the areas that release oxytocin, and to the neural networks involved in forming and maintaining social bonds, as well as in feeling and expressing love and mithra, disrupts and destroys our relationships. Interestingly, neurostimulation by rewiring our neural networks may restore those bonds as they were pre-injury. This has implications for both reconciling and grieving.

Mary-Frances O'Connor in *The Grieving Brain* notes that forming attachment bonds via the nucleus accumbens activates related genes and leads to permanent epigenetic change. As neurostimulation and neuromodulation regrew neurons and rewired neural networks in me, I noticed that some aspects of my pre-injury self, including attachment bonds, re-emerged as if they'd never been disrupted. I theorize this happened because my epigenetics guided that regrowth.

What may happen is that while brain injury remains untreated, we cannot yearn for people who've left us. Our nucleus accumbens as well as our insula and/or anterior cingulate cortex (involved in feeling emotional pain) may be injured and unable to activate. We know intellectually but cannot feel it physically. At an unconscious level, social isolation releases cortisol. But when neurostimulation begins to restore those areas, yearning hits. Our bonds become re-established, guided by our genes and epigenetics as I theorized; it's as if they had just left us instead of years earlier. I found this change confusing—why did I not miss them, then, seemingly out of nowhere, begin to miss them terribly? The regrowth brain biofeedback stimulated in bonding- and emotion-related brain areas may explain why.

Relationships Are Two-Way Streets

We evolved to relate to each other in person. But anyone on social media or the phone has experienced the same feelings as when in person. Perhaps to a lesser extent, perhaps not as deep, but that may not be a function of the medium—in person versus virtual—so much as the duration, frequency, and depth of the interactions. After all, pen pals in times past formed deep, lasting bonds. Our brain maps the closeness dimension of each person we interact with, and mirror neurons activate regardless of the medium of connection. I wonder if these neurons also activate when we read another person's thoughts through social media, heightened by accompanying photographs, GIFs, images, or video? We hear their words in our minds and see their thoughts through their images or GIFs. We observe their emotions changing under social media peer pressure similar to when people rally together on the street, in clubs, or in homes. When we read their tweets or Facebook comments, we directly gain their cognitive perspective, a part of empathy.

Our brains can connect to each other no matter the means—in our thoughts, emotions, spirit, and behaviour. In person, on the phone, or virtually. And because our brains activate under any social connection, we can maintain, grow, and be supported in our relationships no matter the means as long as we connect regularly and deeply.

Do we want genuine relationships?

The pandemic taught society that busy-ness had actually created superficial relationships. Human beings need dependable friendships. Mithra holds us together for our physical and mental health. But every time a friend claims busy-ness, they deprive us and themself of activating the mirror neurons and releasing that feel-good hormone oxytocin. They deprive themself and us of learning about each other, supporting each other during good times and bad, and rewarding each other's brains with a hit of oxytocin.

Relationships are two-way streets. Mirror neurons infer the idea of people needing people to thrive. We cannot mirror another if they're not present. Similarly, our nucleus accumbens cannot strengthen attachment bonds when the other person doesn't connect with us.

neurophysiology alone doesn't determine the depth of relationships

Scientists have only just begun unearthing what neurons and other brain cells do to create, grow, and maintain friendships. Philosophers and writers have thought and written about love, friendship, and mithra for millennia. Theoretical physicists study how the universe, and we as part of it, hangs together. Religious scriptures are at their heart about God's relationship with their creation, human beings, Earth, and the universe. As Oprah likes to ask, "What is your intention?" What is your intention towards a loved one when you choose not to spend time? What is their intention towards you when they find reasons not to call? You can't control another person and make them like you, spend time with you, support you, and allow you to support them in whatever way your injured brain permits. Intention speaks to our souls, knowing one is loved enough to have time for the other...or not.

Brain function, trust or distrust, beliefs, attitudes, effort, intention, and love built upon mithra determine a relationship's depth and resilience.

Mithra and love find a way to reach in to a hurting person, persist through adversity, encourage another with no expectation of reciprocation, and has nothing to do with sex or romance yet can become more intimate. That may be what scares people the most about mithra.

CHAPTER 10
———

RECIPIENT OF LOVE

Brain injury lands us in a vulnerable position, as dependent on others as a child or even an infant. As much as children need the giving, self-sacrificing love of a parent, so did we when first brain injured. Every brain injury is different, every sequela unique yet typical. You may be less dependent or more dependent than others with similar injuries. But we all need more care than the average adult. We need continual, non-judgemental love, being reached in to our physical-, cognitive-, and emotion-damaged selves.

Unable to Love

One of the shameful, horrifying realities of brain injury is it can damage our ability to love. Imagine damage in those areas that produce oxytocin or contain mirror neurons. We wouldn't physiologically be able to mirror what we see others say and do. We wouldn't physiologically feel the reward of hanging out with a friend or talking to a sister, brother, mother, or father. Worse, brain injury may also damage the emotion centres of our brain, leaving us without affect.

Affect

Affect is like what we see on people's faces as they experience joy or sadness, anger or laughter. Lack of affect leads to a blank face or unresponsive body language and monotone speech like a drone with a one-tone voice. We may still have the intellectual capacity of love, knowing we love our mother or our friend as we chat with them over coffee or a beer. We may still know what emotions we're supposed to feel. But we present only a blank face. People find that difficult to deal with. One therapist informed me I didn't love my husband because she misinterpreted my lack of affect as lack of love. Talk about doing harm because of her not wanting to learn about brain injury!

Your brain's inability to love does not reflect your loving nature. It only reflects the damage to your brain. The amount of love you feel and can express reflects only the extent of the damage, not your side of a relationship.

Remember: the brain controls everything, so damage to it can affect anything and everything, including the ability to feel and express love and mithra that binds us together.

Yet regardless of how damaged our emotions and affect, or our ability to feel and express our feelings, we remain in mithra with all humans.

Action Plan: Your Brain Injury Reality

One day, I reluctantly agreed to meet a new friend whom I'd only spoken with on the phone. I'd gotten used to her voice, releasing my brain's resources to laugh and chat in real time. But I didn't know her facial expressions or her body language; I knew meeting with her in person would be like meeting a stranger. It was.

With trepidation, I agreed to meet her at a local Starbucks at a slow time of the day. I decided beforehand to order a coffee drink and maybe a small snack to feed my brain since conversation hoovers energy out of my brain. Fewer people around us, fewer distractions, I hoped.

I rested up beforehand and used my home audiovisual entrainment device to enhance my thinking brainwaves. We met outside, went inside to order our coffees, sat down at a free table, began to talk, me woodenly, her as normal. My brain churned through incoming information and stimuli, leaving me unable to respond in real time. Balancing the myriad auditory and visual distractions, her unfamiliar facial expressions and body language in real time, and respond in real time, was like walking a tightrope fraught with falls. Unfortunately, eating and drinking distracted me from hearing and speaking. And like a shy cat, my returning affect hid in the face of seeing familiar people in new situations.

I soon saw she was not happy. Her eyes said, "What happened to her?! The woman who chatted easily and laughed spontaneously on the phone? Who is this non-responsive person sitting across from me?"

I thought, *That's me, stuck with damaged affect and shut-off emotions, taking in your facial expressions as if I'm a baby learning a new skill, unable to speak in real time nor emote.*

She felt my non-responsiveness was personal, even though I'd warned her beforehand. Our friendship sputtered, revived, and nosedived into an abrupt end.

Your Brain Injury Reality

Health care professionals in neurorehab or community care understood and looked past my peek-a-boo affect and damaged emotion centres. They made talking with them easy because I didn't have to worry about what they thought about my expressionless face, my lack of responsiveness. As they became familiar to me, my brain used fewer resources to interpret their voice, facial expressions, and body language and released resources to respond in real time, to express myself closer to normal. They treated me the same, no matter what my brain injury allowed.

Before starting this Action Plan, gather your *Stress and Grieving* notebook, a working pen, set your reward for working on it, and determine which stress buster you'll use to counter the inevitable grief this Plan may bring up. Deep breathe for two minutes. Now turn to a fresh page in your notebook and write at the top, "What Is Your Reality?" Underneath, list or free write your subconscious thoughts.

How does your affect and ability to bond present itself?
- Do you show the world a blank face?
- Can you feel happiness when you're with a familiar person?
- Can you feel good when you're with a new person?
- Do your emotions come and go, mostly off but sometimes they turn on as if launched like a rocket ship?
- Do you show only anger and meltdown?
- Do you feel love or know only intellectually that you love your spouse, your mother, your father, your friend?
- Do you feel connected to other people—do you feel mithra?
- Do you wish you could feel and respond to people like you used to?
- Can you hold a natural conversation?
- What impedes your ability to converse? Think about stimuli, distractions, and familiarity like:
    - A noisy environment;
    - An outside view versus looking at a wall or people when in a restaurant or café;
    - Being at home versus being at a friend's versus being in a café;
    - Drinking while talking;
    - Alcohol versus non-alcohol;
    - Eating while talking;
    - Snacks versus lunch or dinner;
    - Number of people—is it easier one-on-one or with two others than with several people, whether family or a familiar friendship group?

○ Your health care professionals versus your social circle—list each and how you are with each.

Now that you've brought to light your brain injury reality, tell yourself: **These things are what the injury has done.**

This is not a reflection of who you are as a person. Since the brain controls everything, any damage can affect anything and everything from physical and mental abilities to emotions, social bonds, and feeling and expressing love and mithra. Internally, we desire to be with friends and family. Externally, our affect blinks on and off. Some days we're aware of mithra or feel friendship love when we see our friend, other days not so much.

Remind yourself that when someone loves you and shows it, you appreciate it even when your brain injury won't let you show or feel it.

Healing the brain means healing these things. Healing your neurons means restoring your mirror neurons and oxytocin-producing brain cells. It means healing your ability to feel, create, and maintain love and all social aspects of life.

Healing Changes

Without qEEG, evoke potentials, and SPECT scans, we can't see what's happening in our limbic structures, parietal and frontal lobes, and mirror neurons and oxytocin-releasing neurons. We don't know what's happened to them.

Neurostimulation therapies restore these areas rapidly. When affect has been off for years, its return may overpower. Like smelling a super fragrant rose for the first time, we may reel back from the onslaught of emotions. Internal chaos erupts as our brain and self struggle to relearn what's normal while neurons regrow and re-harmonize in a dance of reconnecting and disconnecting until one day they reconnect permanently.

Repeated exposure teaches our brain where to regrow and how to reconnect—and allows returned affect to no longer overpower our senses. Continual internal change generates panic at the slightest external change, for too much change overwhelms. Rapid regrowth feels out of our control. Complicating this brain state is that trauma destroys trust in others and emotion loss destroys trust in ourself.

How can we re-establish relationships with broken trust?

How Does Brain Healing Affect Your Emotions?

This section particularly applies to those receiving neurostimulation therapies or using at-home devices, such as audiovisual entrainment. Start a new page in your *Stress and Grieving* notebook and title it, "How Healing is Affecting My Emotions."

- How is your healing brain changing your affect? Your ability to feel and express any kind of love? Your emotions? Are you aware of mithra—do you feel interconnected with others?
- Do these healing changes panic you? Make you feel like you're standing on shifting sand? Overwhelm you so that you cannot cope with any changes in your external world?
- Are you able to express how the healing affects you?
- Do people believe you? Or do they exclaim, "This is wonderful!" without helping you navigate the chaos from rapid brain changes?
- How do you feel about their lack of understanding?
- What do you want to say to them?

Sharing Your Healing Emotions With Your Therapist

Therapists or psychiatrists who bias towards the DSM lens over the brain-based lens may attribute your outward appearance of your inward chaos to a DSM personality or mood disorder category instead of the actual source: your injured and healing brain. They may not see chaos from rapid change as a problem or respond only with "be positive" talk.

(The DSM or *Diagnostic and Statistical Manual of Mental Disorders* is in its fifth edition, last updated in 2018 by the American Psychiatric Association.)

Choose wisely which of your health care providers is most open to thinking beyond the bounds of accepted medical and rehab practice before you share this section and your answers. You want their help to navigate the chaos and cope with so much change, not tell you to "be positive." If you weren't positive, you wouldn't be attending neurostimulation therapy appointments or reading this book! Prepare first before you share:

- Write a script. Use calm language and practice out loud in front of a mirror. Take your time with this.
- List what you need from them to help you navigate the chaos in your head so that you can function in daily life.

LEARN MORE

> If your health care professionals understand "chaos" as a mental disorder because of their DSM-based lens, give them printouts of the neurophysiological explanations of brain injury, how chaos occurs when neurons vibrate out of harmony with each other, and how they communicate on and off as they regrow and reconnect. https://concussionisbraininjury.com/education/
>
> The cycling on-and-off of a function, emotion, or cognition stops when the neurons, neural networks, and supporting structures complete their regeneration. See https://concussionisbraininjury.com/education/what-is-brain-injury/#why-emotional-trauma-is-hard-to-treat

Remember: these changes are about your brain injury and don't reflect who you are as a person, no matter how others judge you!

CHAPTER 11

UNLOVED

Definition of Unloved

Unloved has many countenances. A loved one encourages, socializes, cares about you before your brain injury; afterwards, they judge, label, reject, abandon, and/or traumatize.

Loved ones justify unloving by using words to characterize you negatively, words like "lazy," "malingering," "anger issues," "depressed," "not getting help," and so on. They define not getting help as not seeing health care professionals they approve of, even when such professionals only dispense medications and use DSM labels to misidentify brain injury as a mental illness. If you can't find a health care professional who treats brain injury as an injury, who reject ordering qEEG or SPECT and prescribing effective neurostimulation treatments, what's the point of banging your head against ignorant specialists who refuse to learn—other than keeping family and friends happy?

Some family and friends justify unloving us by complaining we hadn't acknowledged the stress our brain injury had caused them. But relieving their stress is why brain injury rehabilitation programs and psychiatrists ask to meet with family and friends. Health care professionals teach them about brain injury. They provide support, guidance, and resources much better than we can.

It's a bit much to ask us with brain injury to attend to others' needs while our injury interferes with remembering tasks like brushing teeth or paying bills. How can we offer enough stress relief to make them feel better when we can't relieve our own stress? We're aware of our loved ones' stress and distress, but we struggle to function and cannot meet their needs without neurostimulation and neuromodulation therapies that dramatically heal. We cannot feel better ourself until we're healed, so how can we help them feel better?

Have You Been Unloved?

"They entered my narrow hallway as I returned to my buns in the oven, trying desperately to hold two things in my head at once: the baking buns and the unexpected people at the door. The boys were elsewhere playing with Lego, my parents at my kitchen table. I wanted to go back to the front door. *No, stay by the stove!* I'd realized years earlier that if I let my thoughts wander me out the kitchen, things burned. I had to stay by the stove where the timer would penetrate the cotton wool wrapping my senses and thoughts.

They shouted down my long hallway, "We haven't had lunch. We're going to get Swiss Chalet and bring it back here."

My broken neurons fired chaotically. *I'm a vegetarian. I can't stand the smell of meat in my home. I'm OK with it elsewhere but not in my home. I have buns to bake. Are they baked yet? No, people are at the door. I have to feed them with only eight buns. But they're bringing Swiss Chalet in. I can't have chicken in my house.* The smell memory wrinkled my nose.

Brain-injury anger blasted out my mouth. "No!"

"We haven't had lunch," they bellowed back. "What's wrong with bringing Swiss Chalet in?" They continued that they didn't expect buns. They turned up to visit me.

I didn't do well with no warning. I began to spin around. *Do I have food other than buns to feed them? Good Friday is about buns.*

I'd invited them over for buns.

They'd said no.

Why are they here? All of a sudden? And not wanting buns?

I can't feed them.

"You have to be flexible!" came the shout down my unlit hallway.

I yelled back from the oven, "You didn't tell me!" My brain injury anger was throttling me. *I can't burn the buns. I can't under-bake the buns. I don't know what to do.*

The door banged.

They'd left.

Half hour later, I found their cell number and apologized for yelling. They told me I'd traumatized Freny. My stomach hollowed. My chest burned. My brow furrowed: *No! I didn't want to do that to her! How could I have? But they said I had.* I hung up, no reciprocal apology made, their words whirring in my head until my reason returned. I wrote an email. I feared confrontation. Hated it. But I made myself sit down at the computer. I wrote. I edited. I stared. I edited. I sent to all."

From Concussion Is Brain Injury: Treating the Neurons and Me.

In my email, I attempted to clarify the brain-injury-caused changes in me and what I needed from them to ensure we all had a good time. Only my mother responded. "Good message," she wrote. That Sunday, Freny skipped up and grabbed my hand. She grinned up at me. I hadn't traumatized her. I was relieved yet hurt and flummoxed about why they'd lie to me about that.

Being Unloved Starts With Lies About You

Have people lied about you? Intimated you've traumatized others? Declared you a failure, a loser, unfit to be around others? Have they turned your brain injury into personality defects, scoffed at your inability to keep a clean kitchen or wipe down your microwave? Have they demanded you have a drink with the whole gang, like you did before your brain injury? Then because drinking alcohol worsened your brain injury symptoms, and because brain injury made socializing with more than one or two friends impossible, they found reasons to no longer invite you out? Did they refuse to learn about brain injury, how to accommodate it so you and them could have a good time together?

Did they talk about how your brain injury consumes their lives, while ignoring they leave your brain injury when they go home? Did they not notice you never get to leave your brain injury?

I Tried to Leave My Brain Injury

Back in 2015, I flew to England to visit London and my oldest Aunt and escape my brain injury. My neurostimulation therapies made this rare trip possible, but I still needed help to plan and book it. My peer mentor organized me.

My photobiomodulation therapy doctor treated me to have as much energy and good brain function as possible while away. I packed my home audiovisual entrainment and cranioelectrical stimulation devices. I'd need to use them daily to keep my neurons harmonized under the demands of travel. I created lists and scheduled every part of my visit in my phone's calendar. Under the guidance of my peer mentor, and with a letter from my neurodoc, I arranged for airline support.

receiving regular medical care is a job without vacations

I used to travel a lot before my injury. Brief trips within Canada. Longer, planned trips to the Yukon, the USA, the UK, and Europe. But after brain injury, except for one trip with my mother to England in 2002 and a couple of weekenders to Ottawa to stay with relatives, I'd stayed home. This England trip was like reclaiming my old self. My family was angry. They demanded I prioritize visiting them before I travelled to England. Why? They regularly travelled on vacation, yet I could not? My first vacation in 13 years could only be to them? Medical care is a job. Living with brain injury is constant work. We need vacations, too, from the things that distress us. People who have unloved us distress us.

Unloved isn't only about being rejected and abandoned, it's also about being told what to do to make them happy, to let them stay in denial about their role in our relationships and unhealed brain injury. They focus on their feelings, not doing things to heal our brain injury so that our collective life can return to health.

Accommodation, the Opposite of Unloved

By the end of four days in London, England, I admitted I couldn't escape my brain injury. By the end of my trip, it didn't matter. I'd experienced being treated like a human being whose needs weren't a big deal to accommodate and who was a joy to be with.

My English vacation opened my eyes to the many small injustices back home in Canada, like family and friends informing me they'll communicate with me only in their preferred way, not in the way my brain injury demands; or being given gifts based on who I was, denying the damage brain injury had inflicted on my talents. My English friends and relatives accommodating me happily threw into stark contrast how being unloved had distorted my healing and relationships.

being unloved stabs our heart, twists our guts, shatters our mind

We cannot understand how before our brain injury loved ones invited us over for dinner, answered our call for help, showed mithra in many little and big ways, then afterwards spewed words like "toxic," demanded apologies from us, and claimed we need help when we've lost count of the number of health care appointments and exhausted all help that standard medical care is prepared to offer.

Unloved by Physicians and Therapists

Almost universally, I found health care professionals compassionate and caring. Yet they resisted learning about better and newer ways to help us their patients and clients. As the decades rolled by, I became less and less tolerant of such stagnant thinking. My father is a world-famous gastroenterologist who modelled to us kids excellence in patient care and clinical research. When I began university, Dad and I would stride every morning to campus while he taught me about the art of medicine and good clinical science.

I learnt from my father what excellent patient care comprises and how research informs patient care and vice versa. Decades later, I established the Dr. KN. Jeejeebhoy Award in Gastroenterology at the University of Toronto for a gastroenterology resident who exemplifies the best of patient care—combining clinical expertise with patient-informed research. I grew up thinking all doctors were like Dad: when he had no answer to a patient conundrum, he'd say, "I don't know," then scour journals and colleagues to find an answer. His patients comprised the sickest, and he formed a team to care for them. Every health care professional has a role; his patients improved on that stable foundation of teamwork and innovative care.

That doesn't happen with brain injury care.

Doctors are happy to let us languish. Teamwork is a concept, not a reality. The entire thrust of modern medicine is based on the idea behind "compliance." If we're not thriving, it's our fault for not obeying our doctor. It's not their fault—they're too busy to read multiple journals or one; to enroll in continuing medical education topics that broaden their knowledge about neurons, qEEG, and neurostimulation; to recognize our suffering deserves a practical healing answer—not a few minutes of compassionate listening with instructions on strategies, rest, and positive thinking. Those don't regrow neurons and neural networks.

Being professionally unloved occurs when brain injury specialists and family physicians refuse to learn about neurostimulation, won't order diagnostics such as qEEG that inform treatment, and won't collaborate with the health care professionals who specialize in these areas. Being professionally unloved also occurs when rehab offers only subjective questionnaires, which you and I would heartily throw out the window if we could!

Action Plan: An Instance of Being Unloved

As you read my unloved story, one of your own probably came to mind. Sophie Hannah, a British crime writer, wrote *How to Hold a Grudge*. She developed a system of processing grudges to heal her childhood trauma and continuing wounds. The first step in her grudge-healing system is to write down the grudge. I'm going to adapt her method.

Prepare

Sit in your quiet space, choose your stress buster and rewards for starting and completing this Action Plan, and deep breathe for two minutes. May this space allow you to write whatever comes to mind with no one judging you or limiting you by looking over your shoulder.

Select your *Stories of Healing* notebook. Think about the story of being unloved that immediately came to mind as you read my story. What would you title it?

The story I quoted earlier was about the Good Friday when brain injury anger erupted. I'd title my story, "Hot CROSS Buns." I capitalize cross because cross in British English means angry, but the word in the name of the buns means Jesus's sacrifice on the cross for us. I was trying to give to my family by baking hot cross buns for them. The ones who'd unloved me set me up for failure, and my brain injury anger erupted. The double entendre of the title breaks up the tension and puts the story in a healed perspective.

LEARN MORE

> Brain injury anger flashes on and vanishes instantly. It differs from other kinds of anger in its internal feel. It comes about only after brain injury. "Researchers have failed us, for they've had since the famous case of Phineas Gage[†] in the late 1800s to study anger unique to brain injury that arises out of neurophysiological damage. And

specialists have failed us, for they've not learned from Phineas Gage that it's a direct result of injury, not behavioural or psychological change." See https://concussionisbraininjury.com/education/anger-and-perception/.

Write Your Being Unloved Story

Write your story title at the top of a fresh page in your *Stories of Healing* notebook.

Now write the story of being unloved. Don't think, just write until nothing is left in your head. You may find that the story isn't coherent. It zig-zags all over. That's OK. That's your injured brain finding its way to what your subconscious wants to show you. When you get there, you'll recognize it as it appears on the page under your pen or pencil.

if you're unable to handwrite your unloved story, type it on a computer or tablet, whichever is easiest

I find I get to the heart of my story when I don't pace myself. Instead, I build in rest time afterwards. When I set a timer and plan breaks to conserve energy, I lose track. After every break, when I return to the story, I have to start all over again. Pacing while writing ends up consuming more energy than sticking with it until I feel deep down that the story is done.

Let Your Story Rest

Let your story rest for your usual processing time. That could be 48 hours or two weeks or overnight or one hour.

Once you've processed it, return to your *Stories of Healing* notebook. On a fresh page, write all your feelings and thoughts. Scan your body to describe your physical sensations as well. We cannot heal wounds we're unaware of. We become aware by describing how they manifest in our body and mind.

On a new line, write the words, "It happened."

We wish it hadn't happened. We spend hours and decades wishing we could return to the time before our brain injury, wishing that we still had our family and friends in our lives. You wish this story you just wrote hadn't happened. But wishes don't change the past. As Hannah wrote:

"Understand that you cannot change the past, or other people...it is pointless to argue with reality. If I decide that I can't accept *that*—the bare, bald fact that it happened—then I'm trying to argue with an inarguable fact, which is the most pointless activity in the world."

It will take time with your injured brain to grasp that accepting the fact of it happening is not the same as seeing as acceptable their wounding thoughts, words, and deeds.

If writing isn't enough to help you become fully aware of what happened and to process this story as having happened, then try painting, sketching, or drawing it. Slip the image in among the pages of your story. You may also want to try listening to music that best matches how you're feeling or think you feel. Music, like art and writing, can bring catharsis.

Rewrite Your Being Unloved Story

Now rewrite the story, putting in what you would've liked to have said. Add humour, either in the way you write the story or perhaps adding in your own sarcastic or eclectic way of looking at things. If your sense of humour remains AWOL, attach pretty or humorous stickers on the pages next to what you said or did or doodle over what they said to you.

Lessons

Write down all the lessons you learned from this story.
- What did you learn about the others in the story?
- What did you learn about your brain injury?
- What did you learn about your emotions and thoughts?
- What did you learn about how others treat you?
- What did you learn about how you react to mistreatment and how you'd like to react instead?

Write down any other lessons that come to mind.

remember: you are not your brain injury ➤

You are worthy of being loved because God created you; the universe gathered together photons and electrons, atoms and molecules, to coalesce into you. You're needed in this universe. Other humans don't have a say in whether you should exist or not. God and the cosmos have already shown you should.

Can You Reverse It?

I don't know if you can reverse being unloved. That's reconciliation work. Relationships are two-way streets. Brain injury steers us higgledy-piggledy on our side of the street as we labour to meet the other side. But we can't force our loved ones to meet us, nor is forgiveness reconciliation. Healthy re-loving requires completing the triangle of remorse, forgiveness, and reconciliation.

Sincere, complete apologies heal wounds. Forgiveness from us bridging towards remorse from them, acting out our mutual desire to reverse being unloved and live in mithra, is what leads to reconciliation in friendships and family. More on that in Forgiveness Is Not Reconciliation.

CHAPTER 12

UNEXPLAINABLE ENCOUNTERS

A Chance Encounter

I sat on the waterfront park bench, watching waves lap under the sun, eating my muffin. A duck waddled over to demand his share. I shook my head. He waddled around the bench and snuck up from under me. Oblivious to the blonde woman sitting at the other end of the bench, I remonstrated the duck, "No. You're not getting any." Undeterred, the duck stared at my muffin, its bill peeking out near the side of my leg. I said again, "No. This is mine."

The woman burst out laughing. She'd been wondering who I was talking to when she'd glanced down and spotted the duck. People don't normally speak out loud in public to the ducks demanding their share of our sandwiches, cookies, and muffins.

I smiled back at the blonde woman and told her about the greedy beggars with wings and webbed feet, the sparrows that hop this way and that to catch falling crumbs. That began an hours-long conversation on our bench near the sparkling blue-grey water of Toronto's waterfront under the scorching sun. I didn't want it to end. It was a rare moment of me being visibly liked, of conversing on diverse topics without being judged, and of sharing deep and harrowing moments. Afterwards, she connected briefly on LinkedIn, sending me an encouraging note.

I remember the warmth of this unexpected encounter, our laughter, her complete acceptance of me, feeling like my pre-injury self had revived to inhabit me.

This was a moment of mithra. The glue that bonds loved ones and strangers together, that makes us human. Supportive, sharing, encouraging, growing ideas together, healing, laughing, being silly together. That it came from and with a stranger and lasted only hours reflects how core mithra is to our human nature.

Action Plan: An Instance of Stranger Mithra

As you read my chance encounter story, one of your own probably came to mind. You may have struck up a conversation with a stranger on a park bench or in a coffee shop or, perhaps, your new occupational therapist. Health care professionals come to know you. But they're also like strangers because rarely does the client-therapist relationship develop into a two-way street type of relationship, the kind we have with good friends and loving family members. Still, we're connected through mithra.

Prepare

Prepare for this Action Plan by using deep breathing and your stress buster of choice.

Settle into your quiet space where you can write freely whatever comes to mind where you need not fear another judging you from over your shoulder.

Grab your *Stories for Healing* notebook.

Think about the chance encounter that immediately came to mind as you read my story. What would you title it?

I'd title my story, "The Duck Who Introduced Me to the Blonde." Following Hannah's grudge-healing method, I use humour or quirky words in the title because humour reflects and recreates the story's good energy.

Write Your Chance Encounter Story

Write your story title at the top of a fresh page.

Now write your story without thinking until nothing is left in your head. You may find that the story isn't coherent. It zig-zags and detours. That's OK. That's your injured brain finding its way to what you really want to say. When you get to the end, you'll recognize it as it appears on the page under your pen or pencil.

If you're unable to handwrite, type your story on whatever computer or tablet is easiest. Either pace or build in rest time afterwards, whichever lets you immerse yourself in that wonderful memory as you write.

Let your story rest for however long you need to process it. That could be 48 hours or two weeks or overnight or one hour.

Write Your Feelings and Thoughts

Once you've processed it, return to your *Stories of Healing* notebook. On a fresh page, write out all your feelings and thoughts. Try to describe your physical sensations as well.

<u>*what happened, actually happened*</u> →

Although this is a good story, reliving it may make you cry. In a world of pain, the rarity of a good thing hurts because of its very rarity and because you want so badly for that kind of encounter to happen again. We yearn for people who unloved us to treat us as we were treated in these chance encounters.

Next, write the words, "It happened."

Yes, this good thing really happened to you. Amongst all the people judging and rejecting you, someone came along and said in their words and body language towards you, you're a good person and worth spending time with.

Your injured brain will take time to grasp that healing insight. Dr. Phil once said it takes one hundred "atta-girls" to counter one "bad girl"!

Reinforce With Art

If writing isn't enough to help you process this story as having happened and to become fully aware of what happened, then perhaps paint, sketch, or draw it. Slip your artwork in among the pages of your story. You may also want to listen to songs or instrumental music that best reflects how you're feeling or think you feel. Music, like art and writing, can bring catharsis.

Lessons

Write down all the lessons you learned from this story.

- What did you learn about how strangers see you?
- What did you learn about mithra and how you're interconnected with all humans?
- What did you learn about your brain injury?
- What did you learn about your emotions and thoughts?
- What did you learn about how health care professionals treat you?
- What did you learn about how you react to being treated as a normal person?
- If your reaction wasn't what you'd have liked, how would you have liked to react instead? *Note*: When you consider this question, remind yourself that this pleasurable encounter actually happened, and it remains a good thing!

Write out any other lessons that come to mind. Remind yourself you are not your brain injury. You are worthy of being loved because God created you; the cosmos gathered together photons and electrons over time to coalesce into you. You exist in mithra with everyone else. You're needed in this universe.

CHAPTER 13

HOW DO WE GET TO FEELING WORTHY OF LIFE?

Self-Comfort

We begin our journey to healing by digesting the totality of our brain injury, being unloved and loved, and facing up to the things that grieve us. Denial sustains us through the shock but not over the long term of recovery.

A compassionate voice asks, "Why are you crying?" I hope Step One is helping you answer that question.

Counter the Unloved Stories

Return to your stories. For every unloved story you wrote in Action Plan: An Instance of Being Unloved, write a countering Being Loved one, following the same steps. Your brain injury journey isn't just about being unloved; it's also about the times unexpected people loved you, including family or friends in an odd moment of loving support or when acquaintances, who meant little to you before your brain injury, stepped up to the plate to accept you in all your brain injury glory.

A Being Loved story is like a glaring spotlight on the unloved moments in your life, exposing grief, yet diminishes their message that no one likes you. It revives knowing you're loved and part of mithra.

Repeat this countering step for the rest of your unloved stories when you can. At the very least, counter the unloved stories that replay in your mind and marked your most important relationships. Spread the writing out over weeks or months so that these rare moments don't paralyze you in grief or cause your subconscious to reject feeling and processing grief. As your tears flow out, they carry with them stress hormones, cleansing your body. The act of crying releases oxytocin and endogenous opioids (endorphins); it's why you feel better when you let go.

I know, I know, you're sick of crying! Me too. Crying in the shower, in bed, on the couch, in your dog's ruff. But hopefully now, you're starting to know why you're crying and who you're crying over. Crying is our brain's way of expressing, processing, and letting go bit by bit the ones we loved, our pre-injury beliefs about our relationships, and who we were. I'll talk more about Grief and Healing Grief in Steps Three and Four.

Healing Moments in Nature

"[Judy Taylor opens the Bible and] turns the thin pages to find her favourite passage. Romans 8:31–39 promises her that nothing will separate her from God's love—not her scarred body, not her pain, not her ill health, nothing. Just like God never forsook Jesus, He will never forsake her. She thinks again of that long-ago Friday. Although God's plan was for Jesus to die, He still mourned his death, darkening the skies, rumbling the earth, and rending the curtain in the temple. She feels death hovering near her. She prays again for God to take the cup away and to restore her life, for death not to be His will for her. She shuts the Bible and puts it back in the drawer."

From Lifeliner: The Judy Taylor Story.

Lifeliner was my first book. Judy Taylor lived for 20 years without eating. She was a medical pioneer in artificial feeding, a technology my father developed in Toronto for home use that saved tens of thousands of lives around the world. I had finished the research and started the writing when brain injury stopped me cold. I needed to heal my injury to finish writing it and fulfill my commitment to Judy's family. Yet I drew knowledge and strength from her story for my healing. In the end, I only needed to regain the cognitive foundation of relaxed focused attention, relearn to write, and receive human help, to finish writing the book. After I published *Lifeliner*, my neurons continued to heal as I accessed various neurostimulation therapies when I could afford them. I delved back into fiction and wrote books, screenplays, plays, and essays.

You may find as you go through the Action Plans that you have more Unloved Stories than Being Loved ones. In that case, every time you write or reread an Unloved Story, reread one of your Being Loved ones or model Judy and read a passage from scriptures about how God loves you. Ask for the peace that only the Creator can provide, the kind that flows into the whole of you and lets you weather a difficult situation.

Nature also reflects how we're all equally small in the universe's vastness, how we're a part of our planet, and how our species interacts with the flora and fauna of our world. We all came into being in the same way. No one person is worth more than another.

Seeking Healing Moments in Nature

Artificial light tries to hide the universe from city dwellers. But I've discovered that even in Toronto, in between too-bright streetlights, I can see the stars. Those few stars reassure me of how I'm a part of the universe's immeasurable magnificence.

From your window or a nearby park, if it's safe, look up at the sky, the moon, or the stars until you feel and know you're part of the universe, as small and worthy as all other human beings. Researchers discovered that standing near a tree confers a sense of calm. Plants, dogs, and cats do the same. Pets and Nature give our sanity a break and remind us that even when rejected by all, a being and forces greater than all humans put together, love us. Nature reminds us of mithra—how we're interconnected. Nothing exists in a vacuum. No species is an island. All of us are essential.

God does give us more than we can handle because we are social beings, created to live in relationship, a network of humans holding and giving to each other in mithra. But when brain injury or a pandemic comes along, we see that we've created a society that counters mithra and Nature's or God's intention. We end up alone.

So what do we do?

RELATIONSHIPS

Given to us

For us

So

WHY

Do they leave?

Step Two

RELATIONSHIPS

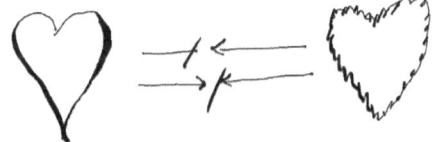

CHAPTER 14

RELATIONSHIP WITH OURSELF

How Does Brain Injury Damage Self-Love?

I was washing my hands at the bathroom sink when I glanced in the mirror. My hands stalled. I stared into brown, glittering depths that stared back at me. Who was that? Not me. I averted my gaze hastily and finished washing my hands.

Our closest relationship is with ourself. To thrive, dream, and follow our dreams, we need to love ourselves as we love others—as a person worthy to exist, with a purpose and a role to play, welcomed in society. That's why when the "ourself" we love dies under brain injury, our grief differs from other kinds of grief. We've lost the person closest to ourself.

the brain manifests us, and so injury can kill off who we were

Each brain injury is unique, like every brain is unique. Today, almost 8 billion individual and unique brains work hard to keep alive the bodies they inhabit and minds they're connected to.

Every Brain Injury Damages the Relationship to Ourself Differently

An injury, from viral to car crash, can damage one part while leaving another intact. That leads to unexpected problems amid seemingly normal functioning. It feels like you're lopsided. And forever angry or devoid of all anger. That abnormal anger state disconnects us from ourself.

The neurophysiology of brain injury anger eludes complete understanding, but one perspective says that when the very front parts of our brains are injured, that allows a deep, primitive part to act unchecked. The amygdala reacts to people and situations like an unthinking, cornered animal. Normally, the very front part of our brains, the prefrontal cortex, starts developing and reaches full maturity in our early twenties. That helps us during our growing up years to learn how to interpret facial expressions, body language, to navigate different types of situations so that we stop reacting without thinking and start responding without excessive anger or rage.

Compounding this lopsided combination of losses and retention is an inexplicable worsening of function after appearing to get better. It's like chunks of ourself fade, flare back, then vanish while we remain unaware microglia are behind the vanishing. (See What Is Brain Injury? A Synopsis.)

Can Neurophysiology Findings Apply to Brain Injury Changes? A Theory.

As I read *The Grieving Brain*, I pondered how research findings applied to losing ourself and brain injury grief. Perhaps the brain map of ourself in the posterior cingulate cortex no longer matches the person we see in the mirror, the way they look, the way they move. And so they look like "not me!" But unlike when a person dies and we attend funerals to provide our brain with external proof that the brain map needs changing, our death provides confusing external cues and doesn't shift our attention to the present like funerals do. We see our faces, our bodies; hear our voice, the rustling of our clothes; see others talking to us, not to a photo or gravestone; taste food and smell the flattened skunk; sense heat on our skin and cold on our cheeks.

Our past is our present; the present a distorted future. Our brain doesn't change its belief we will return nor its brain map of ourself to the new person in the mirror. It doesn't shift its attention from the past to the present without proof.

But what happens to our closeness dimension with ourself? How does our brain react when our mind is severed from our brain? Our self no longer exists as a unified whole? Adapting psychologist Arthur Aron's Inclusion of Other in the Self scale, our one circle of total inclusion of self in our self becomes two distant circles of mind and brain split apart.

SELF BEFORE AND AFTER BRAIN INJURY

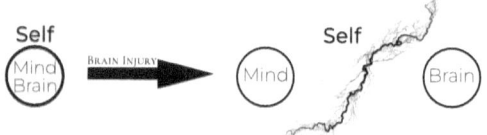

According to Mary-Frances O'Connor, our nucleus accumbens activates and creates yearning in research subjects shown photos of living children or romantic partners. People who experience complicated grief showed greater activation in this region than those in the resilient grief group. We're alive like people in those photos. If shown photos of ourself before brain injury, would we not pine? Would we not yearn so much it becomes physical pain? We do! It's not surprising we yearn night and day for our old self, like our mind is yearning to be made one with our old, healthy brain again, to rejoin its circle of self with the brain's circle of self.

Yearning for Ourself

Brain injury rips our identity out and hurls it into a distant ocean of grief. This isn't a search for identity or purpose; it's a savaging of our core, leaving us asking where we went, who we are. The questions score, gouge, lacerate us day after day. When we receive neurostimulation therapies and stabilize our identity and personality, then we join those searching for purpose.

Like those experiencing complicated grief who continue to yearn for their dead in anticipation of the reward of seeing them again like we do living loved ones, our brains continue to predict the rewarding outcome of seeing ourself again as possible. Don't we find brain injury unreal while seeing ourself again as believable? Only neuroimaging research can prove that conclusively, but it feels like that, doesn't it?

But we know already about some of the changes. Mirror neurons, our emotion centres, brain maps of ourself and others, oxytocin-producing cells, serotonin and dopamine drops—the neurophysiological damage accumulates and changes who we are.

The accumulating losses of skills, talents, and abilities, cognitions and emotions, the ability to read people and converse, the discombobulation of worsening after seemingly better, heaves us back to childhood or lands us in the chaotic throes of adolescence. Fun times, eh?

Brain Injury Mood

Serotonin and dopamine are the neurotransmitters you may know as those being involved in the DSM diagnosis of depression.

But brain injury is not a DSM mental illness. It's an actual injury. Just as we don't fix broken bones with chemicals that flood the entire body, so we cannot fix injured neurons, their supporting cells, and the brain's immune system by flooding the brain with chemicals.

Emotions and mood may feel like they're not physical—for decades, we've categorized them as mental states, divorced from our physical bodies—but they are very much based in the physical brain.

Just as we cannot will a broken leg to walk normally without a cast, pins, or paste applied to the break to rejoin the broken bone, we cannot will or strategize good mood, healthy emotions, and social behaviours without the right treatments to regrow neurons, reboot microglia to repair and sustain neurons, and reconnect our neural networks.

Neurons with short axons regenerate or rewire in no time. But some axons stretch across the brain. Regrowing those, even with neurostimulation therapy speeding regrowth and restoring healthy immune function, takes time. It's like rebuilding a bridge that spans the Pacific Ocean. A healthy brain balances regions working independently with working together. Long axons help with that integration. And perhaps an integrated brain leads to better mood?

Rumination

Like the word "fatigue" doesn't describe the neuro-fatigue after brain injury, rumination after brain injury is not the same as in a healthy person. Rumination is a physical effect of a physical injury, reflected in specific high beta brainwave frequencies of 24 to 36 Hz. Drs. Lynda and Michael Thompson call it "busy brain." It's because rumination keeps our brain busy, occupied with spinning hamster wheel thoughts.

Think of busy brain like a computer processor continually working in the background while you're trying to browse or write or read an email. You can hear the computer processor ticking away, busy on something, you don't know what. Whatever it's working on sucks all the memory and hard drive space so that your apps take minutes to launch and, when launched, respond in slow motion, pausing, ticking away for seconds or minutes, each time you tap a key or click the mouse. A half hour disappears into waiting for the computer as you write one word. The only solution is to reboot it.

busy brain takes you away from yourself

Similar to a chugging computer, busy brain hogs our brain's resources. Not only has brain injury slowed down our processing speed, but busy brain hogs whatever resources are left, making thinking, feeling, talking, listening, walking, etc. slower, exhausting, and tough. Meditation, deep breathing, positive thinking don't stop busy brain—even if temporarily suppressed, rumination surges back. This isn't being anxious or a worry wart. It's a physical effect of the injury to our brain as reflected in high levels of particular brainwave frequencies between 24 to 36 Hz.

LEARN MORE

Only brain biofeedback shrinks or permanently heals busy brain by decreasing the specific rumination frequencies a qEEG shows are the problem. But if you can't afford brain biofeedback, an affordable home audiovisual entrainment device reduces it or frees you from it temporarily. It's more effective than meditation as it targets the specific brainwave frequencies that need enhancing after brain injury: SMR/Beta. These are not the same frequencies as non-injured people need to reduce the anxiety, which meditation works on, alpha and theta. But only a qEEG or evoke potentials can diagnose which frequencies in you need enhancing and which decreasing and where in your brain.

Innate Knowledge of Our Existence

We're born knowing we exist and thus deserve to exist. We form our first relationship with ourself and simply accept ourself as we are. The well-known phrase "love your neighbour as yourself" contains this knowledge. Even though life experiences and abusive people damage our self-love, nothing takes away the relationship with ourself like brain injury does. We no longer know who we are; judged and rejected, we cannot do things that used to come so readily, without thought. Even walking may require conscious thought to tell our legs to move. How does self-love—not self-idolizing nor self-centredness, but the belief that we are worth life, existing, and being with others—survive?

How Others Damage Self-Love

Trauma happens not only from the brain injury cause but moreso from how loved ones react badly to it. When people judge, reject, and abandon us and when they dissuade us from seeking neurostimulation therapies, they injure our sense of self. They damage those parts of our brain responsible for social bonds. They teach us that trust is a lie. We learn not to trust those who profess to love us. We already don't trust the unrecognizable self that stares back at us in the mirror, frightening and confusing us.

Damaging Talk

Being in a relationship with a person who says they love us while at the same time saying:
- "Get on with your life!"
- "Why are you still on the couch?"
- "Haven't you napped enough!"
- "Get a job. You'll feel better."
- "You're malingering."
- "Your child doesn't like you because (fill in the blank)."
- "Why would your brothers or sisters want to spend time with you when you only talk about yourself?"
- "Don't you feel anything?!"

Those statements pierce our heart like rat-a-tatting bullets of bad thoughts and bad words. Like the bad deeds that follow, they damage their target severely. Repair is difficult. Sometimes they fillet vital parts of ourself. They make us feel—and falsely believe—that we shouldn't exist.

other people can induce suicidal thoughts →

Zoroastrianism teaches us to walk hand in hand with God, thinking good thoughts that lead to good words and doing good deeds. The corollary is to resist bad thoughts, words, and actions. Jesus in the Sermon on the Mount reflected this concept when he warned against anger. He wasn't talking about the moral anger over seeing civilians being slaughtered or the bickering over what colour to paint the bedroom or temporary annoyance with good friends. After all, Jesus got fed up with the stupidity of his disciples and flipped the tables in the temple courts when he saw money changers taking advantage of vulnerable worshippers and desecrating God's house. Jesus often sought alone time to recharge and regain God's peace so that he could handle all the pain around him. Jesus isn't a hypocrite. So what kind of anger was Jesus talking about when he said:

> "You have heard that it was said to those of ancient times, 'You shall not murder'; and 'whoever murders shall be liable to judgement.' But I say to you that if you are angry with a brother or sister, you will liable to judgement; and if you insult a brother or sister, you will be liable to the council; and if you say, 'You fool,' you will be liable to the hell of fire. So when you are offering your gift at the altar, if you remember that your brother or sister has something against you, leave your gift there before the altar and go; first be reconciled to your brother or sister, and then come and offer your gift."

From Matthew 5:21-24, New Revised Standard Version.

What kind of anger murders another? The kind that's aimed at you in compassionate tones that speaks the words "we want to help you" or "we love you" but makes you believe you don't belong on the planet. The kind that unloves you and blames you for your mind-killing isolation. The kind that not only induces suicidal ideation but may have driven you to attempt it.

Broken Hearts

Physical changes happen when others break our heart. Sudden, intense pain pressing down on our chest can signal broken heart syndrome. Intense, emotional stress induces broken heart syndrome, from divorce to betrayal to rejection.

The emotional intensity of bad thoughts, of judging, labelling, belittling, and rejecting, snap attachment bonds, break what is core to our natures: love and our heart. Loved ones who want us to deny our brain injury, to act as if we have healthy neurons, to seek mental health help but not brain injury treatments, raise a barrier between us and health. Their words and actions break our core beliefs that when we're in trouble, they'll guide us to help that actually helps. They deny we live in mithra with them, that we belong in our shared community and society. Their words have more power because our brain injury stranded us in an ocean of confusion. They sound so certain that they must be right. We believe their words because we don't trust ourself anymore. Yet somewhere in the depths of our subconscious, we know they're wrong; we know we have an injury and yearn for doctors and rehab to heal us, to restore to us ourself and our place in mithra.

Forgiveness Dictums Compound Trauma

The drumbeat of "you must forgive" compounds the trauma by making us feel even more inadequate, a failure, unacceptable. People telling you to forgive don't help you heal; they reflect societal propensity to victim blame and deepen the trauma to our social bonds.

Jesus's admonition to go and be reconciled to your brother or sister is towards those who unloved us, not to us when brain injury anger erupts. Jesus healed those who were ill and injured, and brain injury anger is an injury effect. He didn't condemn us. He knows the power of apology and reconciliation based in truth.

I write more on forgiveness later in this Step and grieving who you were under Step Three: Grief.

LEARN MORE

> The American Heart Association writes a good explainer on broken heart syndrome. They write, "Tests show dramatic changes in rhythm and blood substances that are typical of a heart attack. But unlike a heart attack, there's no evidence of blocked heart arteries.
>
> "In broken heart syndrome, a part of your heart temporarily enlarges and doesn't pump well, while the rest of

your heart functions normally or with even more forceful contractions." The good news is that most recover fully within weeks. Researchers need to learn much more about it. https://www.heart.org/en/health-topics/cardiomyopathy/what-is-cardiomyopathy-in-adults/is-broken-heart-syndrome-real

Can You Restore Self-Love?

Healing begins with the core knowledge that God and the universe loves you—that your existence is good, you're needed and worth being fully healed. Your brain can be and should be restored to health.

You cannot persevere to grasp qEEG and neurostimulation therapies unless you believe you're worth the soul-sucking battle of self-advocacy and the rewarding, hard work effective treatments bring.

Fighting for effective treatment in a medical system that espouses strategies and rest as the epitome of healing, in a society that treats brain injury as a personality disorder, is arduous and draining. Yet finding appropriate assessments and attending neurostimulation therapies will reward. As injured talents and skills return to life, your self-confidence regrows.

treated neurons restore life →

In thinking about how I endured through years of seeking treatments and resisting those who wanted me to stop, I realized I kept at it because I knew deep down, at an unconscious level, that Jesus loves me. I'm not alone in the battle, and I'm worth being healed. I clung to this knowledge subconsciously when every loved one either denied my injury or fought me or labelled me or abandoned me. Even when I quit—and I've quit for months multiple times—that knowledge reaches in and pulls me back to seeking and receiving actual healing. It's true for you, too.

Self-love crawls back as you embark on healing your brain injury grief and treating your neurons.

Action Plan: Do You Really Not Want Healing?

"My coach directed me to the positive psychology questionnaires at authentichappiness.org, run by the University of Pennsylvania. She wanted me to discover my top five strengths. I did it. My top strengths were creativity, ingenuity, and originality. I felt no emotion. While on the website, I spotted one for optimism and hope. It had few but strange questions. I was rated optimistic. *Cool*, I thought, *I'm more positive than my neurodoc thinks I am. He can't dispute this objective evidence.* He questioned its validity. "I wouldn't be here if I wasn't optimistic," I pointed out. I added that he was the one who had extolled positive psychology. He admitted that, smiling readily. He read out loud the only low score of optimism I had for good events persevering, and I suddenly understood what that meant. He agreed I had a right to be angry about my situation but felt he had advocated for me. "I'd like to try again," he said positively. I doubted it was worth it."

From Concussion Is Brain Injury: Treating the Neurons and Me.

That last thought sounds negative, but it reflected the reality of my situation, trapped between a rock and a hard place.

Was putting the effort in to stay with my neurodoc, to let him try again, worth it? I still don't know. But the alternative was no psychiatric or psychological care. Few medicare-covered therapists treat people with brain injury in Toronto; none in some parts of Canada. The optimism questionnaire's results were right: if I wasn't optimistic, I would've quit years ago.

You're Not Negative

You may have heard innumerable times from many people that you're negative, that you're not trying or you don't want to heal. Loved ones may have dismissed your countering statement that you're realistic. You may have come to believe them.

They're wrong.

I know this because you picked up this book. You still have hope in you, still believe somewhere deep down, or maybe overtly and loudly, that you can recover from your brain injury. You're optimistic enough to continue searching for effective therapy and healing.

Positive Psychology

A few years ago, I connected with a wonderful woman with brain injury who was training to be a life coach. She directed me to Martin Seligman's positive psychology website at the University of Pennsylvania. A year earlier, my neurodoc had bounced in to our appointment, enthusing about a continuing medical education course on positive psychology. And so when my life coach suggested using the website's questionnaires, I thought this could help me in more ways than one.

Reject the Negative Label

What is negative? I think it's more negative to label a person depressed in the face of objective evidence of brain injury than to question standard medical care of strategies and rest. I think it's negative to grip tightly to a DSM label than to recognize both that the label is wrong and that the person has good attributes underneath their unhealed brain injury. It's affirming to question if it's worth it to stay with a loved one or health care professional who refuses to learn.

We must self-advocate in the face of disbelief. Too many snuggle into their assumptions, their comfortable wing chair of familiar ideas and familiar traditional medicine of chemistry and surgery. They disdain lifting themselves out of their comfortable chair and entering the new land of neurostimulation and neuromodulation. Family and friends may believe they see clearer than you because "depression" clouds your judgement. Retorting "I'm not depressed! I'm brain injured!" sounds defensive to resistant ears. Self-advocacy becomes this deadening cycle of defending yourself to people who don't want to change, who don't want to learn about objective diagnostics and effective treatments.

> *you can't change or control stagnant people* →

You can't make them like you by acquiescing to their wrong ideas, either. Backing down and accepting their lies about you slices off your self-worth. Rejecting their lies while guarding your psyche strengthens your self-worth.

You're reading this because you still want to heal despite all the hurling mud bombs and obstacles. You have the power to pursue your healing. Taking the positive psychology's optimism questionnaire will attest to that.

Take the Optimism Questionnaire

You'll find the questionnaires at https://www.authentichappiness.sas.upenn.edu/testcenter. The **Optimism Test** is under the section *Engagement Questionnaires*.

The optimism questionnaire is short. You'll have to create an account with the site, but you'll be able to take any of the questionnaires for free and track your results. We will get to one of the other important questionnaires later in this book.

Remember: this Action Plan is for you. It will inform you about yourself so that you know what needs healing and what is good. Maybe you believe you're optimistic, but after years of being told you're negative, you're not sure. Or maybe you aren't optimistic, and seeing it in black and white will help you reflect on what that means to you. In either case, the results are a step towards treating your neurons.

Print and Reflect on Your Results

After you finish the short optimism questionnaire, print out the results and file them in the *Stress and Grieving* notebook. Return to them as you're able to, to process and reflect on the results a bit more.

For now, turn to a fresh page in your notebook and head it, "Optimism Test Results."

Write in a stream-of-consciousness way all your thoughts and feelings about these results. If you lack affect, focus only on writing out your thoughts.

Reward yourself, and use one of your stress busters to decompress.

Later, when you've processed the results more, write again until you feel that you've grasped the fullness of their meaning for you.

Share Results Only with Supporters

Don't show the results to doubters and haters to prove you're not who they say you are. Only show the results to those who aspire to learn about brain injury *and* who have supported and encouraged you to find modern ways to treat it. You want a supportive response that allows you to talk out the meaning of the results, including over successive weeks or months as your brain slowly processes them.

My neurodoc's response pushed me into a defensive position, the opposite of being empowered. But he learnt a few years ago, after one of my social events that rocked him, that I have good reason to believe good events don't persevere. He dropped the "you're a negative thinker" talk, either because he got dead air or I shot back, "I'm realistic," every time. Even if he hasn't changed his mind, I no longer have to hear it. That's better for my psyche.

CHAPTER 15

RELATIONSHIPS WITH OTHERS

What Are Your Relationships Really Like?

"Family life often changes dramatically after brain injury. Changes may persist for months or years." Brainline.

This book presupposes you're alone in your journey towards recovery, that most or all of your relationships are long gone. You may have family around, but they're not interested in understanding your brain injury, how it's affected you or themselves, and in helping you access full testing and neurostimulation therapies. What do you do then?

What is your relationship really like? That's the first question to explore for each of your relationships, past and present. Drawing a pyramid of relationships may help you visualize where you are now. Your closest and most important relationship is with yourself, so self is always at the top.

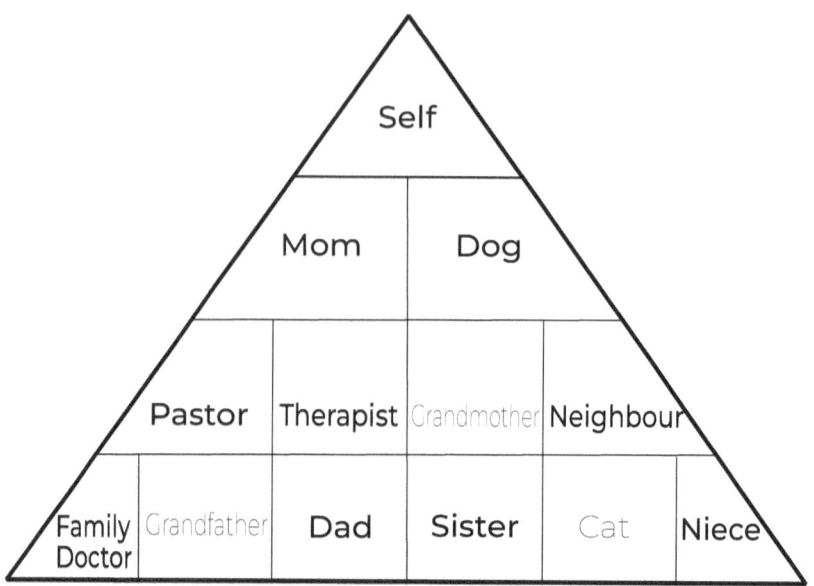

Pyramid hierarchy of relationships. The relationship with self is at the top because it's closest. This example shows Mom and Dog closer, with their more trusting relationship with self, than Dad and Sister. Deceased are in grey text. Dead loved ones still exist in our neural encoding (see Closeness Is a Dimension). It's why we can still have relationships with them, albeit only mentally or spiritually.

LEARN MORE

> Brainline contains scores of informative articles on brain injury, including on family change and how caregivers can recognize and think about those changes. The Family Change Questionnaire helps people understand how brain injury affects everyone in the family. You can find the questions at https://www.brainline.org/article/family-change-after-brain-injury.

Action Plan: Learn Family History

Brain injury destructs your role in your family and friendships. Family history affects how you and your family members react to your injury.

A Snippet of My Family History

"[The] Japanese invaded Burma, causing [my father's] entire family to flee to India in 1942—his father with the army overland and him, his pregnant mother, and maternal grandmother, along with a motley group of refugees, in a Dakota airplane flown by Chinese pilots. As they approached the Burma-India border, the Indian Air Force flew out to fight off the Japanese attackers. He went from a cushy life to an uncertain, nomadic one in India; he determined to become self-sufficient."

From Lifeliner: The Judy Taylor Story.

My parents grew up during WWII. My mother lived on the east coast of England, where as a young child she saw German bombs drop in her rural area, their shapes resurrecting in her mind when she saw the local church's organ pipes. Meanwhile, my father grew up in Burma, safe and secure, mostly an only child doted on by multiple adults, taught by his maternal grandmother. His 18-month-old sister died suddenly in one day when he was four years old. Then the Japanese invaded and chased himself, his pregnant mother, and his maternal grandparents over the Indian Ocean to India, turning him and his remnant family into nomadic refugees. And so began intergenerational trauma.

My parents learnt to be self-sufficient at very young ages. Staying busy is how adults traditionally deal with childhood trauma, and that's what my parents did. Outside of raising us three children, work consumed my father's hours, volunteering my mother's. They expected us to manage our own problems; my mother taught me to be street smart and fight my own battles; my father taught us to achieve. If you want to achieve, you must be driven. That and high expectations, like most Asian cultures, are a hallmark of Zoroastrian culture.

Knowing my family's war and intergenerational trauma helps me understand their unfathomable responses (unfathomable to health care professionals raised here, not having experienced growing up amongst explosions, flaming airplanes, and people being torn apart and killed around you). Although knowing doesn't change my circumstances, understanding at least helps me cope psychologically. I learnt from reading *What Happened To You?* by Oprah Winfrey and Dr. Bruce Perry that the changes war wrought on my parents weren't simply psychological but brain based. War changed their perspectives and their brain function.

What is your family history on your mother's side? On your father's side?

Become Aware of Your Family History

Gather up your tools, prepare yourself with deep breathing, determine your reward and stress busters for this step. Sit in your quiet place and open up the *Relationships* notebook.

Title a fresh page "Family History" and jot down family history events that affected how your family responds to trauma and catastrophic health problems. Include the gaps and how parents' or grandparents' silence in these areas affected you and your family. You can bullet point the events and/or write little stories about them. If your family has had a fairly trouble-free history, write about the worst event and then write your thoughts about having a calm, peaceful background before brain injury hit.

Being able to discuss this with a therapist is the best thing to do. Unfortunately, for me, I needed a therapist versed in cross-cultural practices, WWII intergenerational trauma, and brain injury. I searched for years to find a competent medicare-covered therapist who had some knowledge of brain injury. I had no hope of finding one versed in all three.

What Do You Do When Alone in Trying to Figure Out Your History?

I had long been my own historian. After my brain injury, I continued that habit. I reminded myself of how family history plays out in parental, uncles', and sibling responses in an attempt to lessen their impact on me. It's not me and my brain injury they're responding to—it's their war trauma. Or inherited intergenerational trauma. Knowing how your family history affected parental and/or sibling responses may help you distance yourself from their reactions, to see them not as personal but as the natural outcome of trauma-induced brain changes. And perhaps, it makes you feel that you're kind of all in the same boat, even if they don't want to admit it.

Read *What Happened To You?* if you can. If you struggle with reading comprehension, bookmark and watch videos on *What Happened To You?* Also, historical events coinciding with your family history. These videos may not only help you understand how your family history affected you and your relatives, but also how your own personal childhood history affected your brain injury recovery.

Spot Patterns

As you ponder your family history, look for patterns.
- How do these patterns affect you now?
- How can you stop them from keeping you stuck in brain injury limbo?

Perhaps a therapist or books or videos on breaking family patterns may help you. For me, the only thing that worked was keeping my distance. As I wrote earlier, relationships are two-way streets. And when one side persists in stuffing you in a box that prevents you from healing your brain injury, the only solution is distance or, at least, keeping them unable to affect your health care decisions.

LEARN MORE

> Loving detachment is a psychological method of distancing yourself from harmful relationships while remaining in mithra and not losing your loving feelings towards them. Several health care professionals told me I had to detach from my family; none helped me do that. You may be in the same boat. After brain injury, it's critical to disengage from people who have low self-reflective functioning and mess with your mind. Loving detachment is a method for doing that, as I wrote on *Psychology Today*. https://www.psychologytoday.com/ca/blog/concussion-is-brain-injury/202002/the-how-loving-detachment

Action Plan: Pre- and Post-Injury Roles

We all have a role in our families. Big sister, little brother, only-child-caretaker of parents. What is your birth order? What is your traditional role in the family?

Open your *Relationships* notebook and list your pre-injury roles in your family and friendships. For example:
- Eldest sister, Siblings
- Eldest child, Parent
- Hosts annual family picnics
- The friend who listens, Friend A
- Best friend, Friend B
- Bakes birthday cakes, Friends and family

Consider Your Pre-Injury and Post-Injury Roles

Now review your list think about each of your roles. Do you still play that role? If not, cross it out. If so, place a check mark next to it. Unsure? Write the role down as a header and underneath all the factors pertaining to that role. For example, as a big brother, your siblings still come to you for advice on their latest car purchase, yet your parents deleted you as Executor of their will and made their second child the Executor. Ask yourself, and be truthful, what do you think or feel about the changes in your roles?
- How do you feel about each role change or being removed through being unloved?
- What thoughts come up?
- Do you still feel you have the role?
- If not, cross it out. Later, in Steps Three and Four, I talk about grief and healing grief over these kinds of losses.

What Are Your Roles Now?

On a fresh page, write "Current Roles," and underneath, list all your current roles, including the role(s) you play in your relationship with yourself. For example:

Relationships With Others

- My Health care manager
- My Cook
- My Appointment reminder
- My Encourager and friend

You may find at the end of this exercise, you have no relationship roles other than the ones for yourself. Allow yourself to feel that grief and fear and release the tears. Turn to Steps Three and Four to recognize and heal this grief of being unloved and left to struggle alone with your brain injury. Not belonging anywhere to anyone, or perhaps only with your mother, like so many of us, truly sucks. But you cannot pursue healing when you suppress grief, deny the reality of your aloneness, or stay stuck in wish fulfillment. Futile wishes suck up energy that you could otherwise use to pursue your own goals. More on wish fulfillment later in Wishes Are Not Reality in this Step.

Healing brain injury's catastrophic trail is a slow process of awareness, grieving, accepting, raging, denial, facing up to it, processing, accepting, and gaining courage to focus on treating your brain and going after what you want.

Action Plan: What Were Your Pre-Injury Relationships Like?

Gather up your tools, prepare yourself with deep breathing, determine your reward and stress busters for this step. Sit in your quiet place and open up the *Relationships* notebook. Write the heading, "My Pre-Injury Relationships."

Then think about your most important relationship from the time before your brain injury. Perhaps your spouse or a friend. Maybe your mother. Write the name of that person down as the heading and underline it.

Then write:
- Your feelings and thoughts about the person before your brain injury.
- The feelings and thoughts they expressed about you, through their words and/or actions.
- How often you saw them.
- How often you messaged them.
- How often you spoke to them on the phone or made a videocall.
- What did you regularly do together?
- Who arranged getting together the most? Or was it equal?
- What role they had in your life.
- How did their role in your life match up with your role in their life?
- How important was this relationship to you and why?

Now do the same for each relationship you had pre-injury.

You may find you'll have to do this in several brief sessions as grief and neuro-fatigue build up. Allow yourself the space and time to cry or simply sit in silence as you process your past.

Action Plan: What Are These Relationships Like Now?

Gather up your tools, prepare yourself with deep breathing, determine your reward and stress busters for this step. Sit in your quiet place and open up the *Relationships* notebook.

Start a new page and title it, "Current Relationships."

Remaining Pre-Injury Relationships

Draw a line down the middle of the page to create two columns. In the left column, list the relationships you wrote about in the previous step in the order of importance to you before your brain injury. Number them.

Now go through that list and, in the right column, number them in importance to you now. Put last the ones who unloved you. Take a moment to notice the change in importance. For example, perhaps your mother was third or fifth in importance prior to your brain injury, but now she's number one.

Starting with the one you wrote as number one now, and in *current* numerical order, assess your relationships as they are today.

Write the name of the person and underline it.

Then write:
- Your feelings and thoughts about the person now.
- The feelings and thoughts they express about you, in words and actions.
- What role do they play in your life today?
- What's your new role in their life?
- How often you see them.
- How often you message them.
- How often you speak to them on the phone or make a videocall.
- What do you regularly do together?
- Who arranges getting together? Is it equal initiation? **Note**: because of brain injury effects, it would be normal for the other to plan and organize coffee dates, walks, and so on, the most.
- How important is this relationship to you and why?

Now, do the same for each relationship in numerical order.

You may find you'll have to do this in several brief sessions as grief and neuro-fatigue build up. Allow yourself the space and time to cry or simply sit in silence as you process your present in the past's light. As part of processing, you may want to contrast your answers in this Action Plan to the previous Action Plan. What, if anything, did you learn?

New Relationships

Let's move on to something good: any relationships that came into your life after your brain injury. These people didn't let your brain injury stop them from wanting to get to know you. They naturally accommodate your needs.

Write the name of each new person and the story of how you met them.

- How do they make you feel?
- How do they accommodate your brain injury?
- What is their attitude to your injury and its effects?
- How often do you see them? Talk to them? Message them?
- What is their role in your life?
- What is your role in their life?
- Would you like to see them more often or less often?
- How important is this relationship to you and why?

Reward Yourself!

Reward yourself every time you work on facing up to your pre-injury relationships as they are now, for building up this big picture of your current social life. When completed, give yourself an extra treat and extra chilling-out-and-doing-nothing time before moving on to the next, harder part.

Action Plan: Wishes Are Not Reality

"I'd lend it to kin first, for family is always with you no matter what. It was the mantra I grew up with, the one I adhered to, the one I knew. As I finished Dr. Claudia Osborn's book on June 18, 2001, the day after my holiday ended, I felt the thrill of achievement and thought about how her book spoke to me. Some of the changes in me that I'd revealed to no one because they'd seemed so wrong, she wrote honestly about. She's brave. I could not wait to lend it out, for loved ones to read all the aspects of brain injury that she disclosed so that they would know and understand without me having to speak about them. Speaking was a strange combination of what popped into my head popping out of my mouth, of dead silence as thoughts appeared then got stuck behind the cotton batting that surrounded my mind, and of shades of my old articulateness and rapid speech when I talked about things I knew prior to my brain injury."

From *Concussion Is Brain Injury: Treating the Neurons and Me*. They didn't read the book. Yet I kept hoping for months and years, thinking yet confused over why they didn't, upset they didn't think I was worth the effort.

Wishes Are Futile

One of the things we do a lot is wish. We wish to be re-loved, for a relationship to return or be better. We pretzel ourselves around the loved one's prejudices and judgements to keep that relationship going. Anything to have a social life.

But pretzelling, trying to be what the other demands, raging at the injustice of it all, seeking revenge, drains our energy and keeps us from healing our injury. Ping-ponging between wishing for them to be back in our lives and hating them, keeps us stuck in unhealed brain injury, trauma, and grief. Only physical healing of your brain and their understanding and remorse will truly restore your relationship. But ask yourself: do you want to be friends with someone who judges and blames their decision to abandon you, the person who's suffered a catastrophic injury? Who doesn't resist their bad thoughts towards you and justifies intentional bad words and actions?

Healing Wishes

Take a moment to deep breathe in your quiet place. Sip some water. Prepare your reward and stress busters. Then open up your *Relationships* notebook and start a new page. Title it, "Wishes Aren't Reality."

From the list you created in the previous Action Plan, write the first name of an unloved relationship and underline it.

List your wishes for how you want that relationship to be. Don't hold back. No one will hear or see your deepest desires. Admit to yourself in this list not only wishes for the relationship you want, the roles you wanted but don't have in each other's lives, but also wishes rising out of fury and grief.

Repeat this process for all your unloved relationships when you can, as you can. Some of our strongest post-injury wishes are to go back to the way it was with loved ones, who were a big part of our lives, before our brain injury, before they unloved us. It's like a jagged tear through the heart facing these wishes and seeing them for what they are. And so a little at a time, many small therapeutic doses over many weeks, is more healing than rushing to do it all at once. Dr. Bruce Perry teaches about how therapeutic doses, which can be only seconds long, build on each other to effect healing. I write about therapeutic doses in Who You Were under Acknowledge Losses in Step Three: Grief.

When you've finished writing your wishes for each lost and unloved relationship, you may want to do the same for relationships that remain but cause you pain. These may be necessary or dependent relationships, where the other cares enough about you to remain and support you financially or physically, but they create uncertainty in your life or judge you.

When finished, take a moment to breathe in these wishes. Then breathe them out.

Writing Reality Into Wishes

Write in clear printed letters:

> These are my wishes. They are not my reality right now. I cannot live with the fury-driven wishes. I cannot live with relationship wishes as if they can become true right now. They may become true in the future, but they are not true today. They are wishes. Wishes are like minnows holding back the ocean. Can't be done. When I've treated my neurons, I will revisit these relationships and ask myself if I want to resurrect them. For now, I set them aside. I want to focus on getting better, and these wishes are holding me back.

At this point, add to your lists, thoughts that reflect mithra, the kind that brim over in a loved and being loved relationship, although you don't have those right now. Holding good thoughts towards those who did you harm helps you see yourself as striving to grow, to change your perspective so that your moral anger calms. This step isn't about forgetting or forgiving what they did; it's about retaining your integrity and growing your healing. It's about resisting your own bad thoughts and choosing good words and actions as best you can against the onslaught of brain injury rumination, gnat-like focus, and skittish memory. More on forgiving later under Forgiveness Is Not Reconciliation in this Step.

A Final Let Go

You can now close your notebook and leave the pages with your wishes on them. Or you can rip the pages out that contain all your relationship wishes and destroy them. Some advocate burning them safely. Some suggest tearing them up. Or maybe fold them into little boats and launch them in a pond, river, or lake.

Say goodbye to your wishes and relationships and allow yourself a cry as you do so. **Remember**: tears of sorrow and grief release stress hormones and make you feel better.

Reward yourself and rest up for a day or three or however long you need to process this coming to reality. You've done a powerful thing for yourself! You've gained energy from letting go of wishes.

CHAPTER 16

BOOK OF JOB ON FRIENDSHIPS

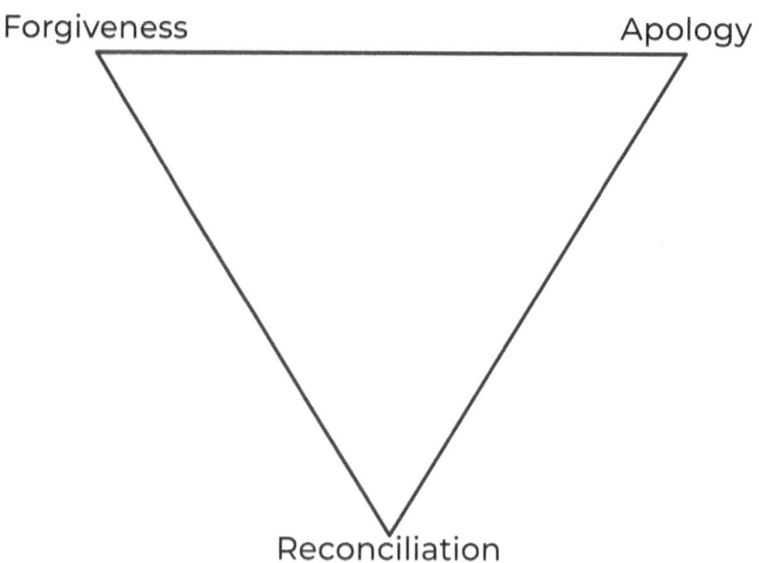

Main Teaching

Assessing your relationships, facing up to your wishes, begins the process of grieving and healing lost ones while the remaining relationships may still be fraught. Religious institutions, ardent Christians, talk shows, self-help books, society—all teach us we must forgive. But putting the onus on us to heal relationships, the ones who were unloved because of injury, causes more harm.

Followers of Jesus know he instructed us to forgive. From secular society, we hear forgiving is for you and about your health, not religion. Rarely, we hear about reconciliation and remorse, the two other points of the triangle of relationship healing.

Former loved ones burden us with another guilt: we must apologize for the ways our brain injury expressed itself and cannot be forgiven until we apologize for our injury. This is nuts. We don't demand a person with a broken leg apologize for limping or for losing their balance and falling against a loved one. The loved one will help right them as they wave away an automatic, "I'm sorry." "You're wearing a cast, you have nothing to apologize for," they'd say. So why demand a fulsome apology for brain injury causing us to fail and fall? Few understand the principle that the brain controls everything so brain injury can damage anything, from thinking to emotions to anger to motivation to communication to walking to breathing. Apologizing for brain injury effects permits loved ones to stick to their falsehood that you're the injury and allows them to avoid learning about brain injury.

If you're still having trouble separating yourself from your injury, return to this Step's first section Relationship With Ourself.

Relationship Healing Is a Triangle of Remorse, Forgiveness, Reconciliation

What people leave out about Jesus' forgiveness instruction is he also instructed that if we know someone has something against us, we're to leave our gift at the altar and go make peace with that person. He also warned that if we—the person who harmed another— do not, we may end up behind bars with the wounded person throwing away the key. Jesus knows relationships are two-way streets. When we've expressed bad thoughts to another, healing begins when we face up to them and act on the good thoughts of remorse and amends.

The Book of Job: An Ancient Text on Friendships

The *Book of Job* reflects that clearly as well.

This ancient book in the Bible is about God making a bet with Satan over Job's worshipping of God. God asserts Job worships God because he loves God, not because God has blessed his life immensely. Satan declares if God takes away everything, Job will stop worshipping God. Ignorant of the heavenly drama, Job and his friends must struggle to understand and deal with his sudden, inexplicable misfortune. Job becomes responsible for God's reputation, for winning God's bet with Satan without knowing it. His friends are tested. Their story is about how we respond to adversity and how we treat the innocent who fall ill. It's about how we treat the least in our society.

> "I read in the newspaper a poignant question, a question we all have when facing the brutal story of childhood rape: 'I don't believe in God,' said the survivor. 'If there was a God, why didn't he help me?'"

This is Job's question. Why do the innocent suffer?

Job was a vibrant and wealthy man, a man of power and influence, a respected man, deeply loyal to family and God; yet Satan, with God's permission, stripped his family and possessions from him and threw him into the muck, as defenceless as a newborn. Not just children are innocent and vulnerable, prey to good intentions and destructive choices. Adults, too, are vulnerable, even ones who look fine on the outside.

Why Doesn't God Help the Vulnerable?

In the 21st century, we nod our heads when we hear "where is God?" and silently agree with the expected follow-up statement: "I don't believe in God." And then when we meet those who've survived horrific childhoods or adult horrors, who say with a fierce love, "I believe," we silently doubt. "How could they?!"

But that is Job's story, told in well-crafted prose and poetry. Misery and unending suffering descend on Job. He laments the day he was born. He likens his life to torrents and calls his friends miserable comforters. Yet he never stops speaking to God. God doesn't answer for many, many chapters as Job grows through his one-sided conversation with God, his thoughts travelling from complaints to wonder about the heavens to his friends to his predicament. At last, in chapter 38, God answers Job. Job again questions, and God again answers. Then Job seems satisfied with God's answers. But God isn't finished.

Job's transformation is our transformation →

God condemns Job's friends and demands repentance before telling Job to pray for them. God instructs what the friends must do and ends with: "My servant Job will pray for you, and I will accept his prayer and not deal with you according to your folly. You have not spoken the truth about me, as my servant Job has."

God has no problem with us complaining about our brain injury and misfortunes. God has a problem with friends blaming us for our misery, complaining, and injury.

LEARN MORE

> I wrote the ebook *The Job Sessions: Why Do The Innocent Suffer?* based on conversations with my pastor, readings, and a group study. It includes handouts and images. You can purchase it at your favourite ebook store for 99 cents.

Who Needs Forgiving?

At the end of Job's ordeal, after God has confronted Job and cured his boils, he declares Job's friends needed forgiving for they didn't tell the truth about God, unlike Job.

Job's friends had put the onus on Job for his suffering. They claimed Job sat in ashes, plagued by boils, because he'd failed, was a complainer, unmotivated. They listed his failures:
- God rejects.
- Stop navel gazing.
- Get over yourself.
- You focus too much on your problems.
- You're not grateful enough.

Do these sound familiar to you? God doesn't like their attitude of casting guilt on the vulnerable. In asking Job to ask God to forgive his crappy friends, God revealed that friends who blame the sufferer for their suffering are in the wrong. Friends who neither sit in silent companionship nor speak comforting words are in the wrong.

Nowhere does God say Job needs forgiving. Only Job's friends need forgiving. The Lord's Prayer includes the words, "Forgive us our trespasses as we forgive those who trespass against us." God forgives the actual bad words and deeds, while we forgive the **persons** who did them. We are neither responsible for their bad words and deeds nor for forgiving their words and deeds.

Wrestling With God or Our Injury Grows Us in Understanding

While his friends remained stagnant in their beliefs, Job processed what had happened to him and worked out his response to losing everything. His thinking transformed from suicidal despair to waiting in settled silence on God. He grew. And when he wrestled with God, he grew a lot.

Wrestling with your brain injury can have the same effect. It can't answer you, unlike God with Job, but it may help you come to terms with it and find your way to healing the physical damage.

friends who blame the sufferer for their suffering are in the wrong

The *Book of Job* shows the sufferer can complain all night and all day long, wish themselves dead, be angry with God, cry out for an advocate, question God, wrestle with their suffering, and grow in their understanding, and God sees nothing wrong with any of that. It makes you wonder if complaining was given to us to process horrendous misfortune, be heard, and seek understanding.

Complaining, like anger, tells us what's upsetting us, gives us a road map out of our predicament when we listen to ourselves. People short-circuit this biological trait when they interrupt us with be-grateful talk, don't hear us out, don't reflect back to us our words to enhance our understanding, and respond without compassion. We short-circuit it when we berate ourselves for complaining, don't listen to the message it's sending us, don't allow a complaint session to end naturally, and do nothing in between complaining. Let the complaint tell you what needs healing. (As your neurons rewire and you heal, your complaint sessions will naturally lessen in number and length.) If you hear anger about judgemental loved ones, follow or review the previous Action Plans. Read *Don't Forgive Too Soon: Extending the Two Hands That Heal* and try the exercises in it. When you hear grief over the loss of yourself, turn to Steps Three and Four to process and heal your grief.

Friends who hold a person responsible for their unjust suffering, who do not empathize with the sufferer, who judge and label and castigate and blame and abandon the sufferer, require forgiveness. See your complaining as God sees it: a gift to drive you towards healing.

For us, busy brain, impaired cognition, absent emotions turn complaining into an endless revolving door; but by listening to its message and treating our neurons, we can progress out of this revolving door, like Job did, and step onto the lifelong path of healing. Look back at each year; see your progress. If you see none, start today!

In creating us, the universe created us the same as all other humans, living and dead. So why do friends or family who judge us believe they're superior and have the right to judge simply because we suffered a brain injury?

A Less Well-Known Teaching

"God once again gives Job seven sons and three daughters. (Seven again, like the seven days of Creation.) But unlike before, when none were named, the narrator names his daughters and only his daughters. Furthermore [unlike for his first set of daughters] Job gives his second set of daughters an inheritance...quite unusual in his patriarchal times."

From The Job Sessions: Why Do The Innocent Suffer?

At the beginning of the *Book of Job*, Job speaks of his daughters in typical patriarchal fashion—as lesser beings.

a perfect and upright man had to suffer to see
the suffering of women and to release them from it

After wrestling with God and God restoring to him all that he'd lost, Job treats his daughters as equals to his sons. His suffering plus wrestling with God taught him that every human life is important. God creates male and female alike as related in Genesis 1. We are all God's children. We are all created out of photons and electrons, the first particles of the cosmos.

LEARN MORE

> "It's strange to me that so many good Christians say that one must not complain. That God won't hear you when you complain. That to 'move forward,' to have God answer you, you must greet everything with a smile. Job puts paid to that monstrous dismissal of intense suffering." Loved ones and therapists make similar demands. I wrote more on this in my *Psychology Today* blog. See https://www.psychologytoday.com/blog/concussion-is-brain-injury/202009/what-is-the-significant-lesson-the-book-job.

Self-Talk

Job talks to God, his friends, and himself. One of the most powerful aspects of friendship is being able to talk things out. We can do that for ourself as well when we self-talk. Job self-talks. He complains about his situation and reminds himself of the beauty of Creation. He defends his innocence, puzzles over God's incomprehensibility, and expresses his grief in all its rawness. As self-talk lessens his anguish, he begins to tell himself what to do.

We can learn from Job's self-talk. Cognitive-behavioural therapy, too, teaches self-talk that embodies good thoughts, good words, good deeds. But it's brief, too brief for those of us with brain injury. With brain injury, self-talk serves many purposes for us beyond what Job modelled. I self-talk extensively. I sometimes wake up having to remind myself what day it is or what I'm supposed to be doing after my weekday morning SMR/Beta audiovisual entrainment session. We can also use self-talk to encourage ourself and ground us when painful memories flash and slash their ways through our hearts and minds. Speaking out loud to ourself about where we are, what we see, what we hear right now reminds us that we exist in the present and pulls us out of those memories. Like Job, we self-talk our steps into healing.

CHAPTER 17

FORGIVENESS IS NOT RECONCILIATION

Resistance Is Not Futile

We don't have to accept blame for the way our brain injury expresses itself.

What Is Turning the Other Cheek, Really?

Christians say to turn the other cheek when faced with aggression. Everyone believes that means to be passive. But it doesn't. First-century scholars dug up this saying's true meaning.

> "'But if anyone strikes you on the right cheek, turn the other also.' Why does Jesus specify the right cheek? Imagine that you are a poor slave in ancient Palestine and your master is facing you and about to strike you. He cannot use his left hand, since it was used only for unclean tasks. Therefore, he must use his right hand. He cannot strike you on your right cheek with a fist or with the front of his right hand, since this would require him

to twist or contort his arm. Thus, in order to strike you on your right cheek he will have to use the back of his right hand. In Jesus' culture hitting someone with the back of the hand was a gesture that had a very specific meaning. This gesture was used only by those in a position of more power to humiliate those with less power. Masters would backhand slaves. Romans would backhand Jews, husbands would backhand wives and parents would backhand children. The message was, 'Remember your place...beneath me!'

"If you do as the passage says and turn your other cheek (your left cheek) and your master must still use his right hand, then he can no longer backhand you. If he hits you again, he will have to use a fist. Hitting another with a fist was a gesture used only between equals. Thus, by turning your other cheek, you have reclaimed your dignity and communicated that you refuse to be humiliated."

From Don't Forgive Too Soon: Extending the Two Hands That Heal.

Turning the other cheek means, in fact, **compelling the other to treat you with respect—as an equal.** It also forces them to see the lie that they are better than you.

turning the other cheek says they are not better than you →

We don't really have a non-violent cultural equivalent to this first-century gesture. But we can learn from it. We don't have to cooperate with humiliation, infantilizing, and blame for the way our broken neurons express themselves. We can resist non-violently. Silence is a tactic I used in my tweens to resist bullies. I discovered it makes people uncomfortable.

Silence Speaks Loudly

Silence says to the humiliator they're not worth responding to; their words and actions are too ridiculous and disrespectful to expend energy on.

When they talk without listening or helping, their words aren't worth responding to.

Silence As Resistance

When someone speaks humiliating words, I reply, "OK." And say nothing else. I simply stare at them. If you're stronger than me, you may prefer to get up and leave without saying a word. I use it like this:

A psychiatrist may speak some nonsense like, "Not everything is due to brain injury." (That statement is demonstrably false in that the brain controls everything. When the patient has a brain injury, a good doctor first rules out broken neurons with objective tests, not subjective questionnaires and opinions; *then, and only then, if tests turn up negative*, they search for other causes.)

When I hear those dismissive words, I reply with silence. My brain injury helps me with that response because my brain chugs in their words, stalls in comprehension, processes, and connects to my speech centres to voice a response like an old dial-up modem. After staring for long seconds, I retort that the symptom had not been present before brain injury.

I assert my decades-long self-knowledge over their knowledge gleaned from five minutes of seeing me.

Buttress silence with asserting your self-knowledge when they haven't done the work to know you and your brain. The work you've done so far and later in this book will grow your self-knowledge and empower you to resist false statements.

When replying solely with silence, I look at the person, trying not to move. When they fall silent, I continue to say nothing and wait for them to speak first. Use your brain-injury-created non-responsiveness to help you stay silent until they speak.

Notes Can Help With Resisting Disrespectful Thoughts, Words, and Deeds

My brain injury grief was slow to reveal itself because I focused on treating my neurons and managing daily life consumed me. When I finally asked my neurodoc outright for help with my brain injury grief, he refused. He insisted I must be positive, a stance I've encountered before in standard medical care of brain injury. This kind of instruction negates my suffering, like Job's friends were blind to his.

To protect myself from being forced into either agreeing or defending my brain injury grief is real. I wrote a note and stuck it near my phone. When we try to defend our state of being, we don't sound like we're advocating for ourself. We sound defensive. People don't respect defensiveness, and they don't listen to it. When my neurodoc spoke words of be positive, I read from my note. I said, "OK, well, thank you very much for your feedback. I will speak to you on___. If [date] is OK?" Then I hung up.

I also used the note to keep anger in check. Although I'd long since healed my brain injury anger through neurostimulation therapies, being unheard still sparks its vestiges. Reading a note out loud and following its instructions to hang up or leave immediately keeps my words polite and delays my anger sparking to life until after I've left the situation.

After I responded a few times with that polite note, my neurodoc agreed to help me with my brain injury grief. He faced the problem of figuring out how because there's a paucity of research and clinical case studies on treating brain injury grief. I knew, though, that partnering with me in this endeavour, we'd succeed. How many psychiatrists, neurologists, and psychologists partner with their patients, though? While expanding, patient empowerment is not the norm yet.

Facts As Resistance

Another way to resist is to continually bring up the merits of neurostimulation therapies. Whenever you're offered strategies and rest or told to be positive, counter with information on neurostimulation therapies. Since loved ones and health care professionals think it's OK to talk down to you, reciprocating with facts feels good. Your confidence will grow and your sense of competence spark to life. You'll need to learn about these therapies, appropriate, objective diagnostic tests, and how brain injury manifests in order to do this with confidence.

LEARN MORE

> My website page https://concussionisbraininjury.com/diagnosis/ covers several diagnostic tests for measuring brain activity and visualizing neural networks. I wrote about my experience with many of them in my memoir *Concussion Is Brain Injury: Treating the Neurons and Me.*

How often have we been at a loss for words when someone declared, "We know what's going on with you!"? You could reply, "I haven't had a qEEG test yet, and the neurologist won't conduct an objective evoke potentials test, so no one knows what's going on in my brain." Or, "I wish I knew, but I haven't found a clinic yet who conducts qEEG tests. With my neuro-fatigue, it's hard. Can you find that for me?" Or, "I want to get well-researched neurostimulation therapies, but I need help finding a certified biofeedback professional. Can you help me?"

Or you may try saying, "Symptoms aren't causation." Or, "Only an objective measure of my brain activity can show which neurons are snoozing and the reason for my neuro-fatigue." Then ask for help to find and pay for a clinic that uses qEEG, evoke potentials, and neurostimulation therapies.

Use Notes

While you're in a calm state of mind and in a good thinking space, compose responses in your phone's Notes app, peaceable words you'd like to use to resist bullying, humiliating, belittling, and rejecting words. Or stick similar notes next to your landline phone or in your wallet. When loved ones verbalize their bad thoughts to get on with your life or be positive, read the note. When your health care professional refuses to help with a brain injury symptom or grief, read the note as your response.

Although brain injury anger has its own timetable, try to stay in as neutral an emotion as possible. The advantage of reading from a note or staying silent is that it helps to reduce the risk of brain injury anger erupting before you manage to leave the situation; it helps to keep your tone even or your affect emotionless. This gives the disrespectful person the message that they're the unreasonable ones and you're their equal and deserve respect.

Forgiveness Is Not Reconciliation

Although resisting will help your self-confidence and keep your eyes focused on healing the brain injury, it doesn't heal the trauma. Continual blame and abandonment worsens brain injury and ruptures our hearts. Yet we're told to forgive the ones who unloved us and health care professionals who abandoned us to strategies and rest.

Forgiveness traditionally includes forgetting while not requiring any acknowledgement of harming us, accountability, or remorse with amends. Bury the wound; pretend an offender had good intentions; wave away any need for an apology because "they had good intentions." We're rigid, resentful, angry for not forgiving their thoughts, words, and actions. Since that's an intolerable way of being, the command to forgive has now morphed into "Do it for yourself."

Superficial Advice Is Unhelpful

One modern attitude: If you hurt, that's on you. Another is: Don't hold grudges. The newest is: forgive because it's good for you and doesn't mean forgetting. Let go to feel better.

Some admit that letting go is hard; some present it as a simple act of unclenching your fist and blowing the ash of the person now dead to you off your palm. This advice feels superficial after brain injury. It centres on us, the one already struggling to make it through the day. Experts don't consider forgiveness's effect on the offender nor about holding them to account. Ancient texts teach a more human idea of forgiveness.

Forgiveness Involves Mithra

The weird part of "do it for yourself" is who espouses it—preachers and pastors, not just talk show hosts and self-help authors. The central message of God is relationship: we're meant to model our healed relationship with God in our relationships with each other. We're meant to see we can only thrive in mithra. How can we hope to gain a restored relationship if the only *reason* we forgive is so we'll feel better? We may feel better about being accepted and seen as "good," but buried wounds create relationships that no longer stand on a solid foundation of trust.

We Are Social Beings

Forgiving only for ourself turns our back on who we really are: social beings who thrive when connected to others. Mithra is essential to our health. So how do we get to forgiveness?

LEARN MORE

> Trauma healers demand we forgive: let go because you'll feel better. Forget, tolerate, or have nothing more to do with offenders. But is that forgiveness? I wrote on *Psychology Today* that healthy forgiveness comprises healing the wound first. See https://www.psychologytoday.com/ca/blog/concussion-is-brain-injury/202110/what-is-forgiveness.

Two Roads To Forgiveness

Two roads lead to forgiveness.
Road One.
1. Heal the wound first.
2. Then wait for the person to return to us.

Road Two.
A. When they apologize honestly, accept the apology.
B. Heal the wound before, during, and after.

In road one to forgiveness, we process the trauma, heal the wound, and then become open to the traumatizing person returning to us in the future with a genuine apology and remorse.

I feel like road two is rare. It's rare a person who blamed and abandoned us for our brain injury will return and apologize spontaneously. Let's talk about that one first.

Healing in Road Two. When the traumatizing person spontaneously and honestly acknowledges to us what they said and did was wrong, expresses true remorse, and asks for forgiveness, their words and actions suture wounds and spark the forgiveness process in one go, if we're open to the possibility. We are social beings. We catch each other's emotions. When the remorse is genuine, we know it. As in A, their apology begins or completes our wound healing, depending on where we are in trauma recovery; we can further heal our wound, as in B. When we're open to receiving an apology, to hearing their sincere remorse and how they will mend our relationship, the barriers the trauma had erected evaporate. When their good words cancel their bad words, they smooth out the scars.

Healing in Road One. Forgiveness begins with healing our wound and is completed while we wait for the traumatizing person to return and are open to their apology.

If we choose to not wait but instead rush the forgiving process—if we skip steps 1 and/or 2—we tell them their cruelty was no biggie; it gives them an out from doing any repair work. In effect, we paper over our wound for their comfort.

Allowing people to experience the consequences of their bad thoughts, words, and actions gives them the chance to grow. Papering over the harm and its consequences in order to obey the command "forgive!" to prove you're an acceptable person, keeps the status quo and buries pain. Both parties must be honest about the harmful event because peace cannot happen without truth. And peace between people is necessary for reconciliation.

What Is God's Wrath, Really?

I don't know why God allowed my life to become a river of losses. Why God watched so many abandon and lie about me. But God and Jesus prepared me to endure and find treatments through my background, education, multiple health experiences, spiritual experiences, talents, interests, persistence and stubbornness, and empathy in order to fulfill their purpose. Like with Job, I wait to see their purpose revealed and met here on Earth or in the Resurrection.

But while you and I wait to see what our brain injury, trauma, and grief will bring forth, how do we heal our wounds as part of forgiveness?

It's important to know one more thing first. In the last book in the Bible, *Revelation*, God's wrath isn't hell or judgement rained down. It's all the traumatized persons' blood, torment, distress, and pain poured out on oppressors' heads, the ones who harmed us and have no remorse. Imagine the overwhelming nature of experiencing our pain, our traumatic wounds, our brain injury all at once! God wants people to feel remorse and act to heal the wounds they've caused. But when they don't, the consequences are to feel it themselves.

God is on the side of the oppressed. Your side.

Is Nature Indifferent?

What about if you don't believe God exists? Norm Macdonald, Canadian comedian, retorted in 2019 to Neil deGrasse Tyson's aphorism that the universe is indifferent to our pains. He tweeted:

"Neil, there is a logic flaw in your little aphorism...Since you and I are part of the Universe, then we would also be indifferent and uncaring...we are not superior to the Universe but merely a fraction of it."

When we scan the detritus of our lives, we feel like people don't care. But Norm is right in his inference that humanity cares; caring drives the trajectory of history. Because humanity does sorrow over our pains, the universe that we're all equal parts of does as well.

Action Plan: Healing Relationship Wounds

I highly recommend *Don't Forgive Too Soon* and *How to Hold a Grudge* for healing relationship wounds, whether you're on Road One or Two to forgiveness. *How to Hold a Grudge* by Sophie Hannah may be a little confusing because of the way it's structured, but her principles are sound. I found these two books the most effective resources to bushwhack my healing path.

Let Go of Expectations

As my spiritual mentor advised often, *let go of expectations*. Easier said than done.

I learnt this skill when dealing with insurance companies. The law works like a hurry-up-and-wait system. You wait for months. Nothing happens. Suddenly, you must rush around signing forms, meeting your lawyer, attending appointments with the insurer's lawyers. I survived this years-long, soul-sucking system by forgetting about the lawsuits during the waiting times.

Fortunately, brain injury includes living in the moment and forgetfulness. Use that feature for your benefit. Once you've finished this Action Plan, file it out of sight (or mail it), and distract yourself immediately to facilitate it leaving your mind. That way, you can't worry about expectations. You're letting go.

Begin the Action Plan

Sit in your quiet space with paper and pens. Exhale out your nerves over this step and inhale strength from the universe. Slow your breathing into deep breathing. Now let's begin.

Write letters to each person who unloved you in which you detail:
- Your hurt.
- What you admire in them.
- What you had wished for them, yourself, and your relationship with them.

- What you realize you need now from them.
- Why you can't continue the relationship as it is.
- How you're going to do things differently in the relationship.

Handwriting the letters, if you physically can, allows your subconscious feelings and thoughts to emerge. You don't have to mail the letters. If you find that they're mostly a tirade (kind of normal), I'd recommend not sending the letters. You can file them away to read down the road to see if you've changed since then—does what used to stoke anger and revive hurt, now not so much? That'll be a measure of your wound healing.

If the letters balance hurt and admiration, include changes you plan to make or have already begun making and why, then perhaps send them and see what happens. But ensure you've given yourself time to think over your words—are they good words? honest words?—and to read and edit the letters several times before you do so. And prepare yourself for any kind of response from silence, to eviscerating criticism, or welcoming and remorse. If you have a trusted therapist, work with them on digging out all your thoughts and emotions and putting them on paper and on deciding what to do with the letters. Mail, file them away, or destroy them as a final act of letting go of those relationships.

Healing relationship wounds is a process; you may need multiple methods and processing over years to get to a place of peace. See the Action Plans in Step Four for further healing the wounds caused by others.

Don't forget to reward yourself for each time you sit down to write or edit the letters.

Forgiveness, Apology, and Reconciliation

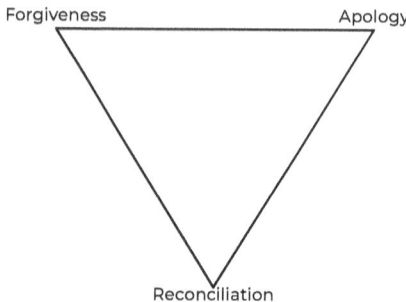

Let's look again at the three-sided triangle of remorse or apology, forgiveness, and reconciliation. When people relate Jesus's instruction on forgiveness, they leave out the full story of how Jesus intended for apology, forgiveness, and reconciliation to play out.

Matthew 18:21-22, New International Version:

> "Then Peter came to Jesus and asked, 'Lord, how many times shall I forgive my brother or sister who sins against me? Up to seven times?' Jesus answered, 'I tell you, not seven times, but seventy-seven times.'"

Jesus then tells a story of a master with servants who owed him debts. The first servant begged his master for forgiveness; responding to the servant's genuine remorse, the master forgave him his debts. But then that servant turned around and demanded payment from the second servant, who was indebted to him. Even though the second servant begged for forgiveness, the forgiven servant refused to accept his request for mercy. The master heard about his hypocrisy.

> "Then the master called the servant in. 'You wicked servant,' he said, 'I cancelled all that debt of yours because you begged me to. Shouldn't you have had mercy on your fellow servant just as I had on you?'"

Furious, the master demanded full repayment of the forgiven servant's debt. Jesus's story asserts our interconnectedness, our mithra, and how forgiveness is tied to remorse in an act of relationship that flows outward into other relationships.

Is Forgiveness Only for Ourselves?

Modern thought states that forgiveness is the way to healing self. It ignores the essential part in Jesus's story: the indebted servants expressing remorse and asking for mercy leads to forgiveness. As we're forgiven, so must we forgive a remorseful person.

Ryan Howes on *Psychology Today*, 31 March 2013:

> "My professor, the late Lewis B. Smedes wrote: 'To forgive is to set a prisoner free and discover the prisoner was you.' Smedes wrote the book *Forgive and Forget* in 1984, which has been credited as the catalyst for modern forgiveness research."

But What Happens After Forgiveness?

Is it enough to forgive? Do we want to ignore mithra, or do we want to restore the relationship broken by betrayal, abandonment, bad thoughts towards ourself?

These questions come up during brain injury recovery because the litany of people who abandon us, the injured, requires a response beyond nightly weeping.

The overriding message to those of us harmed by betrayal, abandonment, and judgement is to forgive—to reward bad thoughts, bad words, and bad behaviour towards us by not resisting, by not revealing them for what they are, as if mithra doesn't exist. Unfortunately, conversation around forgiveness ends at forgiveness and the self: "It will make you feel better; it's about you, not them." But that wasn't the original idea of forgiveness.

Forgiveness Exists in Mithra

> "The root of 'forgive' is the Latin word 'perdonare,' meaning 'to give completely, without reservation.'"

From The Word Detective, 5 December 2007.

One of the most powerful images of forgiveness came 2000 years ago when Jesus from the cross forgave humanity. He didn't forgive to make himself feel better. He sacrificed himself and asked for God to forgive the crowd in order to reconcile humanity with God. In a way, you can say that Jesus was a mediator.

Mediators work to reconcile opposing viewpoints or parties in a legal dispute. The College of Physicians and Surgeons of Ontario offers the option of mediating a disagreement between a patient and physician or surgeon, the idea being that "resolution is one you and your doctor have chosen together, rather than an outcome chosen by a committee."

A Picture of Reconciliation

N.T. Wright, in *The Lord and His Prayer*, suggests "The Parable of the Prodigal Son" in Luke 15:11 could be called "The Parable of the Running Father." What is this running father like?

Wright focuses on the running part. But the father waits for the insolent son to return before he runs to embrace him. This father doesn't sprint after his jerk of a son as the son saunters off to the pleasure dome. The father doesn't consign him to hell nor turn his back on him forever. He doesn't gloat over how natural consequences will mete out accountability to his son.

Instead, this father healed his wound and waited for the son to return as in Road One in the previous section. Ancient teachings reveal the wisdom of waiting, not rushing, to forgive and reconcile.

When the father sees the son returning, that's when he runs to meet him, even though he knows self-interest is still motivating his son.

The father embraces his son *before* the son acknowledges to himself what a jerk he'd been to his father. It's the all-giving embrace that leads the son to see himself, his words, and actions for what they were: abhorrent. At that point, the son repents—he changes his mind about himself, what kind of person his father is, and his perception of their relationship. He changes his attitude from entitled, disregarding of any other human, especially his father, to revelling in his father and their relationship. The son recognizes how much he'd wronged his father.

Return, embrace, repent—apology is a winding relationship path that begins with waiting and returning.

The jerk of a son weeps with gratitude for finally seeing what he'd done, for his father's forgiveness, and for enjoying their relationship in a way he hadn't before. He doesn't seek forgiveness because he's already received it. On the heels of intertwined remorse and forgiveness comes reconciliation.

Notice the father has the strength, health, and healing to forgive unreservedly. We don't have those with brain injury. Mithra allows an unreserved apology to sweep away the pain and bandage the wound. But in the absence of an apology, don't see yourself as less than when you cannot forgive before they recognize what they've done. It's slogging hard work to forgive an unrepentant person when you're struggling with daily life, can't find treatments for your physical injury, and are still healing your relationship wounds. Instead, focus on how the father *waits* for the son to return.

Only Reconciliation Alleviates Isolation

Brain injury isolates the injured person; forgiveness doesn't ease the isolation. Only reconciliation can do that. Forgiveness forms only one corner of a relational triangle, the other two being apology and reconciliation. While apology and forgiveness can happen apart from each other and apart from reconciliation, reconciliation can only occur when both sincere apology and truthful forgiveness are present.

Is Their Apology True Remorse?

Sometimes, the health care professional who didn't educate themselves on how brain injury looks, thus misdiagnosing or making incorrect, hurtful assumptions about us, will try to get by with a quick "I'm sorry my approach hurt you." Even when compassion deepens their voice, this dismissive comment distances themself from the hurt they caused. They place the blame on some abstract approach rather than recognizing their thinking process led to using it. This kind of apology is not rooted in truth. It allows them to avoid responsibility for their bad thoughts that lead to their wrong approach. This kind of distancing won't lead them to a brain-injury-appropriate approach nor confront their possible hidden confirmation biases, weaknesses in familiar therapeutic approaches, lack of listening, built-in antipathy to learning or leaving their comfort zone, and so on.

Another kind of apology by a loved one or health care professional, "I'm sorry I hurt you," sounds like it takes on responsibility. The "I" statement acknowledges that the speaker hurt the person. Yet it, too, belies the truth. By not specifying how they hurt us, they skirt around acknowledging the specific harm they caused. They avoid examining their own thoughts, emotions, words, biases, and actions that lead to harming us.

Their seeming sincerity shifts responsibility for the continuing strife onto us by saying, "I admitted to hurting you, so now you're just holding a grudge." They amplify their past wrong and keep it churning on in the present.

Reconciliation Is Restoration

Just as a furniture maker cannot restore a beautiful cabinet without careful inspection, understanding the exact nature of the damage, and patient, focused work, the wrongdoer cannot restore the relationship they broke without carefully inspecting their own thoughts, understanding the exact nature of the damage those thoughts created, speaking out loud what they did to us and have now learned, and patiently working to incorporate those lessons and rebuild trust.

the person who harmed us bears the burden of reconciliation ⟶

Yes, it's the wrongdoer who bears the burden of reconciliation, for their bad thoughts and selfish actions broke the relationship in the first place. That's even more necessary when it's a health care professional who traumatized us. The first step towards reconciliation is an effective apology.

The Six Steps of an Effective Apology

Christopher Bergland on 13 April 2016 wrote on *Psychology Today* about the six steps of an effective apology, noting:

> "The researchers concluded that while the best apologies contained all six elements, not all of these components are equal. In a statement, Lewicki said, 'Our findings showed that the most important component is an acknowledgement of responsibility. Say it is your fault, that you made a mistake. The second most important element was an offer of repair.'"

When the offender offers to repair the relationship, they're acknowledging that they're responsible for breaking it and thus for restoring it. This is the truth. The six steps for showing they understand their fault are:

1. Expressing regret.
2. Explain what went wrong in their thoughts, words, and actions.
3. Acknowledge responsibility for the wound.
4. Declare repentance.
5. Offer to repair the damage they caused.
6. Request forgiveness.

Notice asking for forgiveness comes last!

In Matthew 5:23 in the Bible, Jesus didn't only tell his followers to forgive; he also told them that when you know someone holds something against you, go to them and reconcile. He taught this after he spoke about facing up to our thoughts and how they lead to actions that harm others.

Therapists cannot tell those with brain injury to go and reconcile. They're working with us the traumatized individually, on our thoughts and emotions. Reconciliation work requires working with both the wronged and wrong-doers. Health care professionals running couples or group therapy can hold the wrongdoers responsible and guide them through the six steps of an effective apology, guide the person with brain injury through the tough process of forgiveness, and bring the two or more together in the intense, patient work of reconciliation.

Brain injury makes expressing thoughts and emotions almost impossible under stress and in real time. A couples or group therapist who gets that and can facilitate expressing your thoughts and/or feelings is necessary.

If the health care professional themself has done the harm, then surely they themself needs to go and reconcile with us, beginning with the six-step apology.

Reconciling With Ourself

Those of us who receive neurostimulation therapies may find our pre-injury self returning in small bits and big pieces. If this happens years after brain injury, conflict may arise between these pieces of the pre-injury self and our changing, present self. Grieving our loss of self, working through regrets (see Regrets in Step Three), help us reconcile the two selves. But it's a dynamic process as our present self continues to change, sometimes suddenly, sometimes gradually, as neurostimulation and neuromodulation restore neural networks and various brain areas. Gradually, the angst of "Who am I?!" fades away. But the work of discovering the new self, with new purpose and new meaning, continues (see Steps Three, Four, and Five).

Optional Action Plan

If you're unsure if you're ready to forgive or even could forgive, the Positive Psychology Transgression Motivations Questionnaire may help you.

Login at authentichappiness.org with your username and password, the ones you used for the Optimism Test. Click on Questionnaires to go to the list (don't look for the test in the Questionnaires sub-menu, it's a bit frustrating). Scroll down to the section titled *Engagement Questionnaires*. Click on the link **Take Test for the Transgression Motivations Questionnaire**.

The **Revenge Motivation Score** may be the most helpful in revealing how revengeful you really are.

I scored below average. I've never seen the point of revenge. That's not to say I don't rage or have fantasies or brief wishful moments of them "roasting in hell," but I prefer using my limited energy to treat my neurons, to do what I enjoy, to read and write. Fundamentally, I don't wish my brain injury on even my worst unloved enemy. That means if you score higher than average on the Transgression Motivation Questionnaire, I have no experience or knowledge to draw on to advise you. I recommend finding a therapist or clergy or a health care professional who can help you work through those legitimate but self-destructive emotions. The book *Don't Forgive Too Soon* may also help, for it talks honestly about vengeful thoughts.

> *Wanting revenge is an understandable state.*
> *Healing it is healthier than acting it out.*

The Challenge of Mithra

Through mithra, humanity reaches our individual and collective potential. God created all of us and loves all of us. Floods drown the revenged and vengeful; noon sun bakes the traumatized and traumatizer. The universe sees no difference between humans when it joins atoms to form our bodies. Revenge goes against the grain of both God's love and the universe's creating force. Our abandonment and isolation teach us to avoid doing the same to others—when we listen to their lessons.

Revenge Ain't Worth the Energy

Those revenged on will want nothing to do with you. That was my reaction when people who I thought loved me used my sudden vulnerability to get back at me for perceived ills. I'm not sure what they thought would happen. Did they think their revenge would make me comply with their wishes? Did the thought of getting their own back feel more satisfying than adapting our relationship to brain injury? Were their bad thoughts and words so ego-boosting they didn't want to question the fears that birthed them? Did they deceive themselves that they weren't being revengeful? I'm unsure they thought about the consequences, contemplated I'd be loath to reconnect, once I'd restored enough of my brain to make independent choices.

An Alternative View

Vengeful words, couched in helping language and compassionate tones, shocked my beliefs into shards that knifed me every time I thought about my loved ones. But their revenge released my energy and time to pursue what mattered to me as the human being God had created—to restore my reading, to breathe through my writing, to discover the mind, and to advocate for decent brain injury care. When ironhearted words broke our bonds, they created an opening for me to craft a new narrative unencumbered by my old roles, to rediscover who God created me to be. The grieving didn't vanish, but the healing sped up.

After being unloved, what does your freed up time and energy allow you to do? Treat your neurons and heal yourself!

GRIEF
Emerges
Out of the
GOOD
and
the *BAD*

Step Three

GRIEF

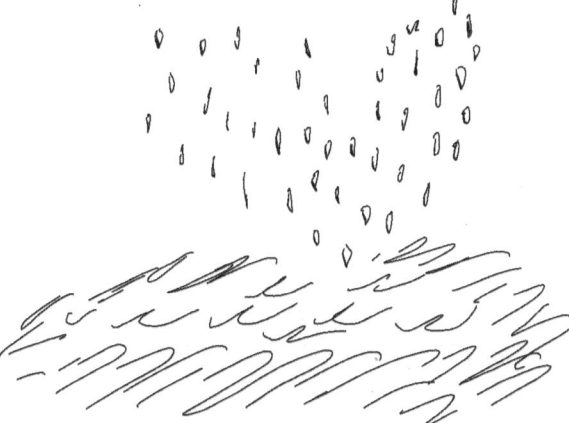

CHAPTER 18

DEFINITIONS

Ambiguous Grief

Ambiguous grief occurs after a loss for which there is no closure or clear understanding. We cry without knowing why we cry. Our hearts bleed tears and our brains emotional pain without knowing why. Our souls find no finality in a grave or certain knowledge that a relationship is over either from death or a mutual parting of the ways.

Complicated Grief

Many years ago, some smart researchers interviewed over 1,500 adult couples and followed them as they aged and became widowed. Mary-Frances O'Connor in *The Grieving Brain* chronicled their findings, starting on page 82. They developed a model of grieving. Almost two-thirds of the couples in their prospective study showed resilience. They grieved, but had no depressive symptoms. About 10 percent had chronic depression before their spouse's death, which continued afterwards. About 10 percent had chronic depression before but improved afterwards. And about 10 percent developed chronic depression symptoms that had not substantially subsided by 18 months, although gradually did by 48 months. The researchers named this last group as having chronic grief.

A group of bereavement and trauma experts convened in 1997 to hammer out the primary symptoms of a grieving disorder. The symptoms are:
1. Yearning for the deceased preoccupies the person.
2. The loss causes traumatic symptoms.

Separately to this, psychologists Margaret Stroebe and Henk Schut, University of Utrecht, Netherlands, developed a model of grieving called the "dual process model of coping with bereavement." Basically, a grieving person lives their everyday life, while experiencing both loss stressors and restoration stressors. They ricochet back and forth between everyday life, loss stressors, and restoration stressors. It's like one moment you're pouring cereal into your bowl, the next you're sobbing all over your cereal, the next you're learning how to clean the kitchen because that had always been your spouse's job, the next you stall over the sink to weep, then you hear the doorbell, dry your face and answer the door for your ride to work, smiling at your co-worker.

We're familiar with loss stressors; we're living in them! Restoration stressors are things like having to learn how to pay your taxes after your spouse, who always did them, dies. At first, you struggle to learn. It feels hopeless; you'll never learn how to fill in the byzantine forms. You storm and rage; sit staring at the tax forms. Why did your spouse have to die and leave you with this crushing burden?! But bit by bit, the forms reveal their secrets; you master paying taxes; and it becomes part of your everyday life.

Yearning

The attachment bond to the dead creates a yearning for them. Nature wired our nucleus accumbens to create yearning in us when we're separated from the person(s) we're attached to. Like hunger and thirst, yearning is a motivation state, designed to drive us towards the necessities of life: food, water, and living in community, attached to other people. Those with complicated grief show greater activation of the nucleus accumbens than those with typical adaptation to grief. More activation equals greater yearning. Yearning creates a preoccupation with the deceased.

The brain requires evidence through our everyday experiences that its physical encoding needs to change, that the attached person is gone. When a person is stuck in complicated grief, they need help to rewire the brain and slowly adapt to their new life without the attached person in it.

> **LEARN MORE**
>
> "although there are shared features between depression and grief, they are not the same. For one thing, there is no specific person or thing that people with depression are preoccupied with, or yearn for." Mary-Frances O'Connor in *The Grieving Brain*, page 124. Read more about how grief and grieving manifest in the brain in her well-written, accessible book.

Feeling Grief

When we stub our toe, nerve fibres send signals up to our sensorimotor cortex, which registers the pain sensation but doesn't give us the qualia—the raw feeling—of pain. The anterior cingulate cortex, which is in front of the posterior cingulate cortex, does. This region directs our attention to what's important and registers feelings of both physical and emotional pain in two separate but adjacent areas. The insula controls autonomic functions, plays a role in regulating the immune system, and is involved in basic survival needs.

When we lose someone, the anterior cingulate cortex co-activates with the insula to create the feeling of suffering. This co-activation doesn't end as we heal our grief, but it lessens. You'll be laughing with friends, watching a movie, when without warning, grief gushes a maelstrom of tears and heart pain. That's normal. But healing grief leads to briefer and fewer of those moments.

DEFINITIONS
Brain Injury Grief

The closest relationship we have is with ourself. Brain injury grief fills every cell with tears when our self dies while we remain alive, aware, and at some level cognizant of the losses.

We don't know who we are anymore.

Losses build up. Abilities, skills, talents, social relationships, hobbies, work, travel, homes, emotions, and/or thinking and communicating abilities—gone. Brain injury grief encompasses ambiguous grief such that the losses are so numerous and cumulative that we may not know what we're crying over or why the psychic pain imprisons us in bed for hours or days or weeks. Closure eludes us; understanding skips away from our grasp.

Brain injury grief encompasses complicated grief, too, yet challenges our understanding more. Treating grief after brain injury as if it's just ambiguous or complicated grief doesn't quite hit the mark. One significant difference is that friends and family typically support a grieving loved one when a person dies physically but don't support the grieving loved one when brain injury causes identity death, not physical death.

I pondered what challenges a damaged brain faces when it loses itself.

Brain Map Loss and Nucleus Accumbens Activation

The brain map in our posterior cingulate cortex no longer matches ourself in the mirror. Yet we lack physical evidence we're gone because we can see, hear, smell, and feel ourself every day. Friends, family, passing strangers, and health care providers reinforce the fact we still exist. Yet our attachment bond to ourself isn't being met because brain injury vanished who we are. Like hunger eats our stomach to motivate us to open the fridge, yearning hollows our stomach and motivates us to hunt for our old self, the one encoded in the brain map. I theorized how our nucleus accumbens would create the highest yearning to fetch our own dead self. And our posterior cingulate cortex would hang on to the belief that we exist exactly as we were before brain injury.

What Happens When the Insula Is Damaged?

A damaged insula may not co-activate with the anterior cingulate cortex; thus, the feeling of suffering may not happen. We attend a funeral, observe everyone around us crying, and feel no emotional pain from grief. That state may happen with our grief for our own death: we feel no emotional pain yet have intense yearning that contradicts our belief we still exist. If our posterior cingulate cortex and nucleus accumbens are also damaged, we may feel no loss either—not for another's death or our own identity loss.

But what happens if your posterior cingulate cortex remains undamaged in the presence of a damaged insula and nucleus accumbens? Would we search for ourself without feeling grief's emotional pain or yearning? And what happens with a damaged insula but unharmed nucleus accumbens? Would that combination create irreconcilable yearning without suffering?

Busy Brain Complication

As I thought further on brain injury grief, I wondered about the effect of rumination on yearning. As I discussed in How Does Brain Injury Damage Self-Love in Step Two, busy brain, of between 24 to 36 Hz, creates perseveration of thought. Imagine the posterior cingulate cortex saying this person in the mirror is not us, we must find us; the anterior cingulate cortex getting our thoughts to fixate on loss of self and co-activating with the insula to create the feeling of suffering; with the nucleus accumbens creating an intense yearning state; and busy brain latching onto this brain-driven need to hunt down the lost self. Busy brain would brood on our death. That would potentiate the yearning and seeking and imprison us in the endless question of, "Who am I? Where am I?" The psychic pain would ratchet up to head-clutching, inconsolable proportions.

After Neurostimulation

Treating the brain injury restores lost functions. An insula coming back online and being co-activated with the anterior cingulate cortex can revive feelings of suffering, made intense after years of not experiencing this kind of pain. It's like a smoker who quits and smells a rose for the first time without smoke clogging up their olfactory nerves. While non-smokers adore the rose's scent, that same scent reels the new non-smoker backwards. They perceive it as a heavy, overpowering fragrance until their olfactory system adjusts to the norm. Similarly, psychic pain turned back on can slay a person. We need support to cope with the tsunami of emotional pain, to grieve our own death or others' deaths as if they're new, until our brain adjusts to the norm.

But even with neurostimulation treatments restoring our skills, talents, metabolism, physical abilities, and so on, who we are will still not match the map encoded in our brain. Yet, unlike people who physically die, we will return from the dead. We have neither evidence we're gone nor are we gone permanently.

We not only have complicated and ambiguous grief, we face a challenge others without brain injury don't have: how to resolve grief of a person who still exists and who, after neurostimulation treatments, may return from the dead but be unrecognizable to our brain?

Quadruple Process Model of Brain Injury Grief

Mary-Frances O'Connor in her book *The Grieving Brain* related the dual process model of coping with bereavement. I thought how it fit yet didn't fit with brain injury grief. I believe the term "quadruple process model of brain injury grief" fits our type of grief better. Like the bereaved without brain injury, we experience loss stressors when friends and family leave us and restoration stressors from having to learn the things our loved ones used to do. But we also have self-loss-oriented stressors from losing core parts of ourself. We exist yet no longer exist. And we have the stress of restoring our brains, of resisting the outdated strategies-as-treatment model of brain injury care and fighting to access effective treatments that restore functionality, skills, talents, and identity.

I realized we cannot heal brain injury grief with just talk therapy. But we cannot heal it with neurostimulation, alone, either. We need both. The next section and the rest of this book is about what worked for me, what I learnt to foster my self-healing.

At this moment, because few acknowledge brain injury grief, no rituals exist for it; since there's a dearth of research on it or clinical programs for it, there's little chance of being able to process and heal it in a safe therapeutic environment. Even though some clinics use neurostimulation to relax a client during counselling, I doubt a clinic exists at the time of this writing that combines neurostimulation with talk therapy for brain injury grief. But don't give up. Let's try helping ourself. Step Three is about unearthing your brain injury grief as the first step on the lifelong path to healing it.

CHAPTER 19

ACKNOWLEDGE LOSSES

Grief congests our heart, and bitterness seeps through cracks in our soul. Decongestants of positive thinking split the cracks wide; bandages of visualization exercises fall apart, soaked in overflowing losses. Shame sidles in, whispering we're only OK if we agree with others' beliefs, ones that clash with our lived experience and our body's messages to us. Brain injury demolished who we were, and we cannot discover ourself nor clear out grief as we struggle alone through activities of daily living.

We may riff off some of our losses in self-deprecating conversations or list them to the umpteenth health care professional, but have you named them and faced them fully yet for your own healing?

Let's begin decongesting grief with excavating who you were.

Who You Were

Words cannot describe the pain of losing yourself, of dying while still alive. It's like a child scratching at a thick oak door. Confidently believing the house behind the door still exists, the child plants their feet into the sandy soil before the door; a keening whine rises from their broken heart, vibrating the air to the farthest hills; fingers scratch grooves deeper and deeper into the wood, faster and faster, their nails breaking. Behind the unmoving oak door, shattered furniture litters the crumbled ground. Thick, green weeds tower among the wood fragments, flinging out prickly seeds, growing more weeds, their prickles burning invisible stings, for no one answers the child's wailing to restore the house and let them back in to where they belong.

"Unpack the Boxes of the New You"

Barely months after my closed head injury diagnosis, my social worker wanted me to unpack the boxes of the new me. An opportunity, she said, like unwrapping gifts. I didn't want to unpack the new me. The old me was just fine, thank you very much.

I saw this new brain injury diagnosis like any injury: you get the diagnosis; you follow the medical instructions; you get better; and you return to work. The idea of not being fully healed—unfathomable.

Me wanting to get on with returning to normal and my social worker wanting to focus on an injury-filled future meant we both failed to acknowledge my losses, especially the loss of myself.

On page 185 of *The Grieving Brain*, Mary-Frances O'Connor summarized two of the neuroscientist Noam Schneck's grief studies at Columbia University on intrusive thoughts. After a person dies, the grieved experience conscious, intrusive thoughts about that person. One moment, the grieved are washing dishes; the next they're remembering how the person died or a regret or a poignant moment. But like with coyotes, the more you try to eradicate them, the more they breed. But unconscious processing, as in mind wandering, leads to less grief. Intrusive, conscious thoughts may distract and upset, but trying to shove them away increases both them and grief, while mind wandering reduces grief.

We can't restore our sense of worth and grab the healing we need until we meet our grief and allow ourself to grieve, knowing grief, though it'll diminish, will companion us always. We let ourself into grief by first acknowledging our losses.

Grief Denied, Avoided, and Interrupted

I don't recall how much I talked about the old me, but my rehab team and psychologist had a better grasp of my present than I did. While I worked hard to heal my injury and return to "normal," my social worker tried to communicate the truth of my relationships; my occupational therapist my inability to read while I stubbornly clutched a mass paperback wherever I went; my psychologist protected me from seeing how supported his other clients were while providing me neurostimulation; and my psychiatrist assisted me in relearning to write. Insurance companies (yes, plural) held back my recovery by requiring multiple so-called independent medical exams and assessments at designated centres. I stopped counting at 15. They comprised health care professionals questioning me over and over about the car crash that had injured me or having me answer questionnaires for hours. Because I'd been through the auto insurance mill before, I knew not to acquiesce to being tested for hours; I demanded they divide my appointments into two-hour blocks. I didn't want them to exacerbate my seatbelt injuries.

listening to your self-preservation instinct keeps you safe →

My pre-brain injury self-preservation instinct survived the crash. But in all those hours and hours and hours over the years and years of occupational, social, psychological, psychiatric, and physical therapy, I don't remember being allowed to grieve, to talk about pre-injury me beyond history taking and a bit of storytelling as a precursor to thinking positively about my then-current state.

Health care professionals denying or avoiding my brain injury grief cost me.

A lot.

I'm still healing my grief.

thousands of therapeutic doses heal grief →

Dr. Bruce Perry in *What Happened To You?* talks to Oprah about how we heal through thousands of therapeutic doses. The dose may be only seconds long. Oprah relates how she's never needed a therapist; instead, she and her best friend Gayle talk nightly. Oprah will relate something painful—a therapeutic dose of seconds or minutes—then their conversation will wander into something light; then she'll return to the painful thing, another therapeutic dose. This pattern might repeat over multiple conversations. Similarly, before brain injury, your friends probably listened and empathized with you, as you did with them, in therapeutic doses without realizing that's what you were doing—healing each other.

brain injury slashes away chances for therapeutic doses →

Unfortunately, when brain injury strips away best friends, we're left with therapists and psychiatrists who only talk to us when we show up to our appointments, who rarely reach in to where we are, who don't seem to have mastered the basics of how friendship heals wounds, and whose time-determined therapeutic doses overwhelm us or who truncate our emotional flow when time is up. During this long therapeutic dose, they interrupt. It's like being cut off at the knees when the therapist wants us to think about a positive thing midway through relating a painful thing, especially when we finally hear ourself speak our emotions after our subconscious took 20 minutes to work through broken neurons to verbalize what we're feeling. Helping people with brain injury requires human resources no one is willing to pay for. And so we have to make do with this kind of friendship substitute.

The Narrow Road of Brain Injury Grief

Jesus said to follow him is to go through the narrow gate of himself and walk the narrow road. It's also an apt analogy of living with brain injury grief. Perhaps you feel the same as me: the narrow road is a tightrope swinging high above a ravine, with crocodiles snapping underneath, snakes twining around the rope and strangling my ankles, predators scratching my cheeks and flapping their heavy wings against my head. Yet I must keep walking forwards to a fog-shrouded destination.

Grieving isn't one and done; neither is healing. Wouldn't it be awesome if it were!

Professionals and public alike are so trained in "positive thinking" that many seem incapable of doing what best friends do for each other—listen and empathize before telling us about what we're capable of now.

So how can we talk about and process our brain injury grief over losing ourself and everything in our life? Let's begin by remembering.

Who I Was

Who were you before your brain injury? I was a laugher. Me and my ex would make each other laugh so hard, I'd end up on the floor, clutching my stomach, crying out, "Stop! Stop!" while he'd collapse on the couch. We'd stop when our lungs demanded air. Sarcasm infiltrated my conversation when talking ideas or politics. I liked to see people smile and laugh and know I'd instigated that. I had a very dry sense of humour, and I learnt pretty quickly that it didn't go over well in an office environment. Consultant work was more my style. I could spend hours poring through computer code to find that one errant semi-colon screwing up my program. I didn't swear. Well, maybe I said, "shit" occasionally. But new friends perceived pretty quickly that I didn't swear and strived not to do so in my presence. They even joked about it, and I laughed at myself. I had a circle of friends I nurtured. If one disappeared for a while, I'd accept that, despite the hurt, and welcome them back when they showed up again. My empathic sense connected to their wounds, my psychology degree added knowledge to my empathy, and I'd use those to understand why they had to leave and self-soothe my hurt. Hours-long phone calls were my jam, listening to friends and family, providing my perspective, giving advice. Listening was my strength, my empathic sense a core part of me, and helping them made me feel an active part of the relationship. Writing novels became my dream. Wouldn't it be awesome to write what I loved to read? I read everything in sight. I honed new skills after I left home, signing up for courses every year after I graduated from the University of Toronto with my B.Sc. in psychology.

*this summary paints a picture of essential me
yet barely scratches the surface of who I was*

My grief is healing. The auto insurance mill and standard medical care denied me telling my pre-injury-me stories for so long that if I began talking about my original me, I'd soon be a puddle on the floor. When alone with no one telling me what I should feel, I used to look at photos and cry. Now, many years later, I avoid looking at photos; when I do, I feel bereft like a dry sinkhole fissuring. I suspect you're as tired of crying as I am, and swallow your tears as much as you can in front of others. So let's in the safety of this book and in your quiet place start to grieve. Know that here you can talk about who you were, in therapeutic doses as long or as short as you can handle.

Action Plan: Your Pre-Injury Stories

Start with two minutes of deep breathing. Prepare your best stress buster to use as you go through this Action Plan, and plan your reward. Find a place where you can sob or stare without thought like we do sometimes or simply sit quietly as your mind wanders through your memory corridors, both fond and painful. This Action Plan is meant to be unfolded, like a long love letter, over weeks and months in therapeutic doses, as you feel ready and able.

Who You Were

In your *Stress and Grieving* notebook, turn to a fresh page and title it, "Who I Was, A Summary."

Start with writing a summary of who you were before your brain injury, like the one I wrote in the previous section. Let yourself feel the feelings. Or if you have no affect, think your thoughts. If nothing comes, let yourself stare out the window as your subconscious processes it. This may be all you can do for now.

Your Pre-Injury Attributes

On another day or time, on a fresh page titled, "My Attributes," list the attributes of yourself that you miss the most. Include abilities, skills, and talents. Include your weaknesses, not just your strengths, moreso if you were working on growing them into strengths.

Your Pre-Injury Stories

When you're ready to continue, return to your summary and reread it to recollect stories about your pre-injury life. On a fresh page, write the first story of your pre-injury self that comes to mind. Give it a title. Following Sophie Hannah's advice about using humour to heal, use something humorous in the title to help counter any bitterness at the loss.

remember the favourite parts of yourself →

When finished, dwell on your favourite part of that memory.

List the attributes of yourself that you liked the most in that story. Then list the ones you didn't like. Write how you changed those attributes as you grew, whether before or after your brain injury.

Feeling your feelings. Knowing your thoughts. How do you feel now remembering that time? List all the emotions. And if you feel nothing, list your thoughts. Let yourself cry or simply sit numb for as long as you need to.

Don't forget to use your stress buster. Other things to help you decompress include hugging a tree, walking or sitting in a park or near plants, looking up at the sky if you have no park near you or garden, photographing flowers with your phone, curling up in a blanket and focusing on its softness, watching the rain.

Whenever you're ready for another therapeutic dose, write another story of who you were.

Recognizing and Feeling Your Grief

When you've accumulated a few stories, return to your first one and read it. How do you feel now? Has your grief begun to surface? Does grief overpower? Or are the emotions of that time returning and the grief abating? That'll tell you if you need to heal the grief (see Step Four) or if grief is healing spontaneously through this Action Plan.

Whenever you want to talk about who you were, write another story about your pre-injury self—or paint or sing or dance the emotions that come up as you return to those times in your memory.

painting, collages, crafts, photography, music, dancing, and walking can help you remember and mourn who you were →

If you have a therapist open to you remembering who you were so that you can grieve that loss, maybe read one of those stories to them so that you can talk about it. Explore your emotions and thoughts with them as a guide. Try to expand on that memory for the duration of your appointment, or across multiple appointments, without them countering your grief with positive talk. The point is not to talk about the now but first to remember and grieve who you were so that you can then heal your brain

ACKNOWLEDGE LOSSES

injury grief and walk with self-worth and confidence into the future to heal your physical injury.

Who You Are

"I forged on, committed to returning to *Lifeliner* in six weeks. The first week of March, my rehab team gently told me I was nuts and suggested I write a newsletter to everyone about my injury, where I was at, my goals, etc. It would force me to confront my reality and give people a clear picture of my situation. I agreed."

From Concussion Is Brain Injury: Treating the Neurons and Me.

Who are you? I mean, right now, as you're reading this? Do you believe that much of who you are is due to brain injury affecting you or a combination of mood disorders, personality defects, DSM diagnoses, and "problematic behaviour"? This section is to show you how much brain injury affects you and expresses itself so that you can discern yourself from it.

When I wrote my newsletter—taking three months to do so—I couldn't believe how long the list was of things that brain injury had changed for the worse in me.

brain injury is not you →

Lisa Raitt, former Conservative MP for Canada, said of her husband with Alzheimer's, "Alzheimer's is not my husband." That's true for you with brain injury, too. Brain injury is not you, yet it has affected you. Describing yourself as you are right now will help you discern yourself from the injury, help you see how brain injury manifests in you. This exercise will hopefully strengthen you to reject inappropriate labelling.

God created you. Nature designed you. The universe flourishes with you in it. Misfortune injured you. But that doesn't make you, the creation, bad.

"The reflective soul does make progress, no matter how limited their knowledge or understanding, while the accuser(s) gets lost in the process of condemning."

From The Job Sessions: Why Do The Innocent Suffer?

Acknowledge Losses

Action Plan: Newsletter

You are what God says you are, what the universe made you: lovable, worthy of love and life. Let's start by discerning what is brain injury in you. I copied the list from my newsletter in the first (2012) edition of *Concussion Is Brain Injury*. I didn't know when I emailed the newsletter that four more years would pass before I discovered the full extent of my losses.

"At the end, the damage included, in no particular order:

- Slow processing (aggravating, and one of the worst problems in many ways)

- Inability to pay attention (think ADD) Inability to focus on one person talking to me in a crowd or group

- Inability to refocus after being interrupted

- Inability to multi-task (it took the "I can do five things at once" old me ages and many mistakes to finally get the message that I was now a "one task only at a time" me)

- Loss of mental flexibility

- Problems with reading and writing (it was years before I fully grasped the extent of these problems)

- Problems with memory

- Problems with communication (e.g., hunting for words, circling around what I want to say)

- Problems understanding others—the more attention required, the worse I got, and no, I often wanted to scream I'm not going deaf!

- Vision loss in one eye that eventually improved so that I can now recognize objects (though very blurrily) with that eye and not just my good eye

- Loss of self ("who I am")

- Olfactory hallucinations (food, usually in the wee hours, just so I can get real hungry)

- Fatigue [now called "neuro-fatigue"]

- Initiation deficit

- Pain (and sometimes feelings of coldness) in the front of my brain, behind my forehead whenever I must concentrate during learning

- Changes in sleep (taking a long time to fall asleep, waking up several times, waking as tired or, worse, more tired than when I went to bed)

- Irritability and anger issues (brain injury anger is not the same as normal anger)

- Vanished emotions (I wasn't just numb, my emotions were gone, except when every now and then they'd fire on violently and take me on a roller coaster ride for about two weeks then disappear again)"

When I wrote my newsletter, only a few months had elapsed since my diagnosis and just over a year since the car crash that had injured my brain. I had so much left to learn about my injury, about the changes it wrought, and about the neurophysiological damage. For you, it may be several years or over a decade or two since your injury as you read this. In that case, you may have trouble discerning between yourself and what you've become familiar with but is actually injury. Learning about typical brain injury effects like loss of concentration, forgetfulness, slow processing, affect, emotional control, neuro-fatigue, and so on, will help guide you. Use my newsletter list as a jumping off point.

This Action Plan began my journey in learning to perceive what was brain injury reality and what was left of myself. Writing the newsletter helped me to resist judgements, criticisms, and DSM labelling as being true.

LEARN MORE

Look at concussionisbraininjury.com/education to become better acquainted with how brain injury expresses itself. What resonates with you? What doesn't? To help you distinguish brain injury from who you are, read up on what brain injury is at https://concussionisbraininjury.com/education. This page comprises the neurophysiology, brain terms, and symptoms. It's not a complete list of symptoms, but it covers the main ones.

Preparation

Begin with your deep breathing and having your favourite stress buster ready. Perhaps set up a small reward for simply starting. Even if you spend only five minutes composing a newsletter, reward yourself. Starting is better than nothing. Repeat the same reward for each time you continue writing the newsletter. Establish a bigger reward for finishing it.

Write the Newsletter

Now turn to a new page in your "Stress and Grieving" notebook and title it "Brain Injury in Me."

Write a newsletter listing your strengths and weaknesses. List the physical, emotional, and cognitive problems you have and trusted people have seen. Use my list above and https://concussionisbraininjury.com/education as a guide to brain injury effects. Write anything that differs from before your brain injury. Include changes in your physical functioning such as heart rate, blood pressure, bladder control, taste, auditory processing, sugar metabolism (diabetes), and so on.

Discern Injury From Yourself

Start a new page, draw a line down the middle, and title the left column "brain injury" and the right column "me." If you wrote your list on a computer, set up a table or use two columns or simply write the heading "brain injury," then after you finish that list, write the heading "me" and write your "me" list underneath.

Under "brain injury," copy from your list what is the same or similar as those in my list above or on the brain injury education web page. Include effects like anger, anxiety, depression, unable to get started on things or complete things, laziness and malingering, the Go button is off (unable to act on thought), diabetes, swearing, emotional control, non-responsive, doesn't laugh, sleeps all day, naps too much, bad sleep. You may also have physical disturbances that I haven't yet written about on the brain injury website such as bladder problems, stomach upset, rapid heart rate, yo-yoing blood pressure, etc. Include all problems that are new to you since your brain injury.

Review that list and reflect on how so much of what people described as mood disorder, anger management, or personality problems are really brain injury effects.

Remember: you are not your injury.

Note that those clinics that diagnose and treat brain injury with objective tests and effective treatments understand brain injury anger is not an anger management problem but a typical expression of brain injury, best healed by treating the injury.

discerning yourself from your injury takes time and multiple tries →

Now write what remains under the "me" column or heading. What's left may include integrity, active on social media, dog or cat lover, ethical, tries to read, keeps searching for healing (aka perseverance), wants to help, relearning, and so on. Because you've gotten rid of all the detritus blocking your perception of yourself, by ascribing it appropriately to brain injury, you may find you'll list strengths and abilities you didn't perceive you had.

#

LEARN MORE

Objective Diagnostic Tests. We're a society that relies on tests to tell us about ourself. Standard medical care uses appropriate objective tests for every part of the body but the brain. This Action Plan may not be enough to help you and others see what is brain injury and what is you. But, I hope, it will give you the knowledge and impetus to demand appropriate objective diagnostic tests such as qEEG, evoke potentials, SPECT, sleep study, and/or diffuse tensor imaging (DTI), which will give pinpointed neurophysiological explanations for why you are the way you are after brain injury. See https://concussionisbraininjury.com/diagnosis for information on these tests. And read my book *Concussion Is Brain Injury: Treating the Neurons and Me* for what they're like.

Action Plan: Your Remaining Skills

Review the two-column list of your brain injury versus yourself. Now let's expand on the "me" column. On a fresh page in your *Stress and Grieving* notebook, write the title "Talents I Still Have."

List all the talents you still have. They may be diminished, and neuro-fatigue and cognitive injuries may have constrained them, but in whatever form they remain in, list them.

Repeat this exercise with your skills and abilities under the titles "Skills I Still Have" and "Abilities I Still Have."

Reward yourself with something small each time you work on this Action Plan. Take the time to enjoy your reward before going on to the next step. You've been honest about yourself, about the actual good stuff. The loss and pain of brain injury consume so much attention that they can obscure the good stuff that's left.

Loss Is Loss but Not Absolute

You want your talents and skills the way they were, not the diminished forms of now. Grief over your losses batters you daily and nightly. But writing out, seeing them out in the open on paper, knowing for certain what survived, reminds you that the loss isn't absolute.

Action Plan: New Gifts Don't Make Brain Injury OK

Let's expand our list of remaining talents, skills, and abilities to include new gifts from brain injury.

My Public Speaking Gift From Brain Injury

Back in 1997, three years before my brain injury, I lead the planning for my fraternity's Regional Meet of the northeastern USA and Toronto chapters. No chapter had hosted a Regional Meet in some time. Organization and planning were my jam. Confidence filled me that my chapter could host this Meet. I lead planning meetings and coordinated booking multiple venues with speakers and events. The only thing I feared was speaking at it. But as leader of the planning committee, I had to speak at the closing banquet.

  I walked up to the lectern on shaky legs. I faced my fraternity sisters and scanned their smiling faces and sparkling eyes. The Regional Meet had succeeded beyond any of our expectations. Blood flushed my cheeks as red as my jacket. I controlled my voice as well as I could and hid my shaking hands. I'd spent hours over my drafts; printed my speech in large-sized font with marks to show me where to pause; reminded myself to raise my head to look over the audience, that my stellar memory meant I didn't have to read with eyes glued to my speech the entire time. But my nervousness over public speaking kiboshed any attempt to memorize the entire speech. Quite frankly, I don't know how I stayed upright! I read my speech fairly well and projected my voice so that all could hear me. My sisters applauded, and I almost collapsed in my chair in joyous relief.

  Fast forward to my first speech after brain injury, also at a fraternity event. My legs didn't shake as I walked to the lectern, expecting the usual agony with the added bonus of gnat-like attention span, no memory, and infinitesimal energy. I figured I could speak for two minutes, tops, and had written the shortest acceptance speech my chapter had probably heard. I laid my speech, printed in giant font, on the lectern, and read it without understanding what I was reading, trusting that my written words made sense. My face didn't flush. I felt no embarrassment, no anxiety. I left the lectern puzzled and awed by my sudden comfort.

brain injury gave me public speaking

After that, whenever I spoke publicly, I'd write my speech at the last possible minute because brain injury had evaporated my ability to prepare ahead of time and only sometimes I had a therapist who ensured I got down to it before the looming deadline drilled into my head I had to get to it. I'd review my speech or presentation just before time, then set it aside. I cannot read and engage with the audience at the same time. I can't comprehend what I'm reading. So I go on memory alone, backed up by my familiarity with the subject, not worrying that my words are mostly spontaneous. Today, I enjoy public speaking without fear.

A rather unexpected gift!

I experienced this gift before I discovered what pre-injury skills, abilities, and talents I had left.

What Has Brain Injury Given You?

Turn to a fresh page in your *Stress and Grieving* notebook and title it "New Attributes." List anything new that the brain injury has given you. You want to focus on new skills, abilities, or talents that lift you up. You may have none or only one. I know how hard it is to admit that such a catastrophic injury has created anything good. I certainly am not grateful for my brain injury, and it's OK for you not to be! But acknowledging or embracing the new gifts doesn't negate the catastrophe.

Spend a little time pondering; don't be afraid to write what comes to mind. Allow yourself the pleasure of discovery, of adding your new gifts to your remaining talents, skills, and abilities. Nourish them in your heart.

A Gift Doesn't Make the Brain Injury Itself Good

Recognizing new gifts doesn't raise the expectation you should be grateful for brain injury. On the contrary, these two Action Plans are not gratitude work. They're about seeing the whole picture of yourself.

With this in mind, pick one of the new gifts you listed and write what you like about it. Write a story of how it's blessed you or about when you discovered it.

Reward yourself and rest up before going to the next step.

Action Plan: Discover Your Top Five Strengths

I wrote earlier about the Positive Psychology **Optimism Test**. Today, let's start the **VIA Survey of Character Strengths**.

Aside from your computer or tablet, the only other tool you'll need is a timer to pace yourself. Set the timer for your standard pacing time. When it goes off, stand up, stretch your body, especially your neck, in the way your physiotherapist or physician has shown you. Look out a window to focus on the far distance, then sit back down to continue. Remember to drink water. Maybe every 15 minutes or half hour or hour, whatever your stamina is, walk to the kitchen and eat something that'll feed your brain. A small cup of organic yoghurt with organic dried fruit and nuts, for example. You want some glucose for instant brain food, but not much, balanced with protein and good fats for slower-acting brain food.

Login at https://authentichappiness.org with the username and password you used for the Optimism Test. Click on Questionnaires to go to the list. Scroll down to the section *Engagement Questionnaires*. Click on the link **Take Test for the VIA Survey of Character Strengths**.

You may have to complete the test over several days, depending on your energy levels and processing speed. When done, print out the results, skim them, and slip the printout into your *Hello Healing* notebook.

Review and Process Your Results

Over the next several days or weeks, return to your results and read the top five strengths and explanations. Notice what the Positive Psychology site says about your strengths. Ask yourself if their explanations resonate with you. Jot down any ideas that come to mind in your notebook. If you cry, turn to Step Four to work through the grief.

good things grieve as much as bad things
after brain injury and years-long trauma ➤

If you have a therapist, take a copy of the results to them so that, under their guidance, you identify and process your emotions and thoughts and discuss any ideas that come up. Your therapist can hold on to their copy as you discuss the results over the weeks, while, with your home copy, you can process them when you're able.

Remember: this is not a sprint but a pilgrimage. There's no rush. Every time you read and ponder, you move a step closer to your goals and heal yourself.

Grief Over Good Things Is Normal

The results may surprise you, overwhelm you, or confirm what you knew. After a few days or weeks, return to the results and read them again. What do you feel? What do you think about them? Review the rest of your strengths, and jot down your feelings and/or thoughts about the strengths not in your top five. It's OK if you find yourself paralyzed with grief. It's normal to cry over good things.

Being alone and unsupported makes pain a constant companion, and good things are hard to believe in, especially when they're about you.

Yes, after catastrophe and years of being alone, improvement and good things bring on grief. Dismissing that kind of grief with "positive thinking" does nothing to help you process and heal it, never mind release you to use and enjoy your newly identified strengths. Acknowledging this grief, and healing it as in Step Four, releases you to feel gratitude and hope.

Accept Being Unloved

Grieving lost relationships and being unloved is so hard that you may, like me, avoid the whole thing. But you can't grieve what you don't acknowledge as having happened. Being unloved runs counter to our neurophysiology. We're made to create and maintain bonds. This feature of our social biology rewards us when we strengthen our bonds in bad times. Our belief that bad times bring people closer reinforces neural networks. Being unloved not only counters our biology, but also betrays our long-held beliefs and societal myths.

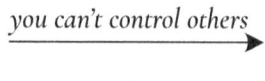

you can't control others

Accepting you can't control others leaves you free to focus on yourself, physically heal your brain injury, and, through neurostimulation therapies, gradually restore control over your own thoughts, words, and actions.

- You cannot go back in time and change the circumstances of your injury.
- You cannot force your neurons to work like healthy ones.
- You cannot restore your pre-injury self so that those who unloved you will love you again.

And, anyway, what's the point of restoring relationships with unrepentant people who so loved you they abandoned you and justified their bad thoughts, words, and actions?

Accepting Being Unloved Is a Process

When my family broke my attachment bonds about three years after my brain injury, they released me from their demands to act as if I had a healthy brain. Having pretty much no affect at the time detached me the next day from the shocking events' effects. The release shifted my focus towards improving my health and away from scrabbling to maintain our relationships. I hadn't realized how much focusing on them, trying to get them to accept the results of objective tests and my brain injury, had given short shrift to my healing.

The release lasted until my affect returned. Then I found it difficult to accept being unloved; I pined for my old relationships. Wishes for what was arose. My wishes landed me back in denying that the break had happened and their unchanging attitudes. No matter how much I told myself I couldn't control them or how much hearing their thoughts about me shredded my self-worth, I still wished.

Facing What Happened Has Happened

A few years ago, I began a conscious effort of using therapeutic doses to acknowledge what happened had actually happened, to teach my brain I cannot time travel and change minds. This process helped my heart work through the grief of being unloved and losing people in my life I'd never thought I'd break from. I accepted that me dying through brain injury had separated us, that their need to deny had cracked wide our separation into an unbridgeable chasm.

I came to realize that not socializing with them allowed me to use my very limited energy to heal my brain and pursue what has meaning for me: reading, writing, and imagining. I've entered the waiting phase of forgiveness (see Two Roads to Forgiveness in Forgiveness Is Not Reconciliation).

Conserving Energy for Healing

Energy conservation is about switching my focus from things that harm me to things that heal me. As long as deniers and avoiders had access to my psyche, they could continue to erode my energy and my self-worth. For someone with extensive neuro-fatigue, that was dire. I had no chance if I chose their feelings over my health, unable to process being unloved over seeking ways to acknowledge this excruciatingly painful situation. Having had years of neurostimulation treatments allowed my injured brain to process it all. But validation and support are key. May this book validate your experience and release you to focus on your healing.

Reputation

Other people control our reputation. Yikes! That's a harsh lesson I had to learn. When someone rags on us, we want to defend ourselves. When a health care professional misdiagnoses our brain injury as something it's not, or diminishes symptoms, we want to get vocal and work hard to get them to hear us. Losing our reputation is not something we could have imagined before brain injury. It's not only part of brain injury grief, it can traumatize as well because it's a relational wound that changes how we and others perceive ourselves in society.

Focus on healing, not defending the injury and explaining how brain injury is not you.

When people don't want to hear and understand, they won't listen to anything you say. Whether you present SPECT scan results or show them qEEG brain maps, whether you talk about your symptoms as appearing only after brain injury or quote supporters, they won't hear you. They want to believe what they believe. It's not for us to understand why they want to think the worst of us or convince us we don't have brain injury; it's for us to focus on our healing.

ACKNOWLEDGE LOSSES

You Can't Change Minds

I've learnt that although people trashed my reputation, overtly lied about our conversations in order to get others on "their side," tried to pit me against others, there was nothing I could do to change their minds. My injury imprisoning me in my head, unable to communicate in real time, hampered my ability to explain. Worse, when I tried to speak the truth, to present facts about my brain injury diagnosis—when I outwardly improved dramatically with neurostimulation treatments—all they heard was defensiveness and the certainty they're right.

don't worry about your reputation →

God takes care of your reputation. "You prepare a feast for me in the presence of my enemies," the psalmist wrote in Psalm 23 about God. But even if you don't believe in karma or God making things right, believe this: put your energy, aim your focus, on healing yourself and treating your neurons. Don't allow others to keep battering you. Protect your heart from their need to vilify, mis-characterize, and judge you. Don't let them drag you onto the treadmill of futile explanations and defensiveness. You have no control over your reputation. I mean, we barely have control over our mouths when injured neurons fire up speech before conscious thinking, so how can we control what others say about us?!

So instead of wasting energy on trying to cajole others to see you, use your energy to heal yourself. And focus on those who support you, lift you up, and speak well of you.

Action Plan: Discerning Responsibility

Thoughts, words, and deeds have consequences. We are not responsible for protecting people from the consequences of their bad thoughts, bad words, and bad behaviour towards us. We do them no favour in trying to wave away those consequences, for denial reinforces their bad thoughts, like how Job's friends kept blaming Job for his hail of losses.

> *protecting people from the consequences of their unloving behaviour damages them and us.*

You've assessed the reality of your relationships and seen that wishes are not reality, and you've worked out what is injury and what is you. But how your relationships ended in the mud may still puzzle you. If you don't know where a relationship went wrong, try this Action Plan.

Where Did It Go Wrong?

As always, sit in your quiet place, prepare yourself with deep breathing, choose a reward for when done, and decide on your stress busters. Take out your *Relationships* notebook and title a new page, "Where Did It Go Wrong?"

This work may be difficult. You'll need to distinguish their actions versus yours versus the brain injury effects.

Go Back in Time. If you kept a dated journal, take it out and flip back to the dates where dark clouds appeared in your relationship and read those entries. Find emails or messages from that time as well, anything to jog your memory. Jot down in your *Relationships* notebook their actions and yours to help you recall what actually happened.

If you don't have these records, write the stories of their first reactions to your diagnosis then their subsequent words and actions that stand out in your mind.

Attitude Changes Over Time. After you've finished writing your stories and/or looking through your records, compare their first words after your diagnosis to later words when the relationship became harmful to you or ended. Record these changes in your notebook.

Either refer to the ebook *The Job Sessions: Why Do The Innocent Suffer?* or the section Book of Job on Friendships in Step Two as you ask yourself: do your friends' and family's words and actions towards you resemble Job's friends?

- Did they at first show compassion and support?
- Did they put a time limit on your recovery?
- Did they blame you for brain injury's effects?
- Did their response to you become same-old, same-old?
- Did they eventually blame you for your suffering?

Your Words and Actions

Review Your Brain Injury Newsletter. Take out your newsletter list to remind yourself of what the brain injury did to you and how it still expresses itself. Review the earlier sections of this chapter to remind yourself of what is you.

- Which of your thoughts, words, and actions have you been blaming yourself for but were really the brain injury?
- Which ones emerged out of your core self?
- Did you change and in what way?

Take a Break to Process

After you've given yourself time, perhaps over multiple sessions, to process and work through this Action Plan, do you see a pattern in how people reacted to your brain injury?

> *Job's friends held him responsible for his suffering, and God declared them wrong to do so* →

And so as the *Book of Job* teaches, you and I are not responsible for others' immature, fear-filled, and repetitious response towards our brain injury. And just like a person with a broken leg isn't responsible for their limp, we are also not responsible for how brain injury manifests.

> "Since we can't undo traumatic events, the only control we have is what we do with it. The more acceptance we can establish over that which we cannot control, the

closer to contentedness we'll be....By knowing what we can't control, we can put more energy into what we can."

From Tyler Henry, Here & Hereafter.

How often have we heard this advice and not acted on it? Maybe rehab taught you the serenity prayer, yet you remained locked in confusion over what happened. The problem is that brain injury takes away control over whatever part is damaged. With diffuse axonal injury like mine, that's almost everything.

What You're Responsible For

I'm only responsible for finding treatment, working with my specialists who are healing me, and keeping myself from harm as much as I'm able to, given the brain injury effect on my memory, neuro-fatigue, cognitive function, ability to stand up for myself, and so on. Exhaustion, neuro-fatigue, and stamina keep interfering and setting us back on our healing path. But have you been diligent in sticking to health care that *has* helped you and in not allowing necessary rest periods to become a permanent stall? Be honest now! If you have been, congratulate yourself. And if not, you're reading this book, aren't you? So you've already taken the first step. Applaud yourself!

> "We must all do our part to live in alignment with who we are and what we stand for....through every hurdle there is an opportunity to learn, internalize, and grow."

From Tyler Henry, Here & Hereafter.

> "My concussion giving me diffuse axonal injury meant it was impossible to live in alignment with my true self. Realizing brain injury took away control over so many aspects of myself, lead me to put my energy into learning about and pursuing treatments that worked. Neurostimulation therapies transferred significant control from the injury back to me. I'm free to start learning about my true self — no longer just the injury — and growing again as a person."

From Brain Injury Wrests Away Control, Psychology Today.

Acknowledge Losses

This self-help book, the website https://concussionisbraininjury.com, and my memoir are the tools to help you find objective diagnostics and attend effective neurostimulation treatments. This book hopefully also complements effective treatments if you haven't had the support and validation you needed to heal your heart and soul.

with brain injury turning off initiation and motivation, you'll need regular support to do your homework

So, while taking responsibility for what you *can* control with support from your health care team—attending effective treatments and doing the required homework—give yourself a break and don't absorb others' blame. I hope you now have a clear picture of each of your responsibilities and how your relationships broke apart. If not, review Step Two and this section, and, as well, check out the Readings section at the end of this book for any books you may find helpful.

Action Plan: What You've Learnt About Relationships

Not absorbing blame and shame is easier said than done!

Lessons From Unloved

Reread your unloved stories. Choose one you can face at this moment. Add at the bottom of it, "I can't control__" and fill in the blank with the name(s) of those who unloved you in the story. Note the ways their unloving affected your functioning and how you felt about yourself at the time. It's really important to see how their unloving words and actions affected your health and your functionality. When others diminish you and exacerbate your brain injury, you can't recover. Give yourself time to process the lessons and emotions before repeating this exercise with the rest of your fractured relationships.

By working through these Action Plans, you're putting in an amazing effort to heal your heart, despite the grief and pain they release. Remind yourself that releasing these losses into the open allows you to process, mourn, and heal them.

Lessons About Your Role in Relationships

Let's turn now to your role. What have you learnt about your relationships? What's the common thread of your role in these relationships *before* your injury? On a new page in your *Stress and Grieving* notebook, write the title, "Common Threads in my Relationships."

List the threads. For example, my main pre-injury one was I set up most of the ice cream dates, dinners over, phone calls—more with some friends than others. My social worker spent six months trying to get me to see that my relationships were me supporting them and now it was their turn to reciprocate, yet they weren't.

Be bold and blunt as you list these threads in your quiet place.

When you've finished your list, leave space to add to it as your subconscious processes the work. Use your stress buster and reward yourself for a job well done!

Acknowledge Losses

seeing the threads of your relationship roles lets you mourn them and learn what to change
⎯⎯⎯⎯⎯⎯⎯⎯⎯⎯⎯⎯⎯⎯⎯⎯⎯⎯⎯→

When you're ready to return, on a new page, write the first thread in your list as a heading. Then, below each thread, write its effect on your post-injury life, especially if your injury impaired or killed off your ability to maintain it. Repeat with succeeding threads.

- Did this thread lead to your relationships unravelling because you couldn't continue it after your brain injury and they couldn't accept that?
- Did this thread lead you to make friendships with people who bolted at adversity?
- Prior to your brain injury, did you excuse unethical, immoral, or non-supportive behaviour?
- Even though you probably heard self-help leaders say to believe people when they show you who they are, did you deny how your loved ones abandoned others so that you could turn a blind eye to it?
- Did you use busy-ness as an excuse to not maintain relationships you otherwise declared were important? Did your loved ones, as well?
- Before your brain injury, did you abandon family or friends who fell ill or were catastrophically injured? Or did you stick by them, and now they've abandoned you?

What has this thread taught you about healthy friendships? What kind of roles do you want to play in friendships and relationships?

Give yourself space and time to feel the grief over this excavating process. It's good work you're doing for yourself!

CHAPTER 20

REGRETS

Regrets can haunt you. Mine centred around pre-injury reading habits and decisions before the car crash.

What Do You Regret Most?

It's late Saturday afternoon. We're north of the city. We drive out of the parking lot and onto Highway 7 after an uneventful periodontist appointment. Moments later, bang! Another dull thud reverberates, thrusts our bodies against the seatbelts. Neurons twist, tiny blood vessels leak everywhere. Myself evaporates, though I didn't know it for several months. For years afterwards, "Why did I go?!" was my constant, silent refrain. *Because you made a commitment*, came the silent reply. My mother had drilled into me that one doesn't break commitments. Period. Rescheduling an appointment if I was sick, was permissible. But that day, I wasn't sick. The day before, I'd overcome a block in writing *Lifeliner*, and I only wanted to hasten back to my manuscript. *If only* I'd put my writing ahead of my commitment to the periodontist appointment! *Then* I wouldn't have been injured! My teeth had been fine!!

Counterfactual Thinking

"Psychologists call our thoughts about what could have happened *counterfactual thinking*. Counterfactual thinking often involves our real or imagined role in contributing to the death or the suffering of our loved one. It is the million 'what ifs' that roll through our mind."

From Mary-Frances O'Connor, The Grieving Brain, page 144.

O'Connor notes that this thinking distracts us from the pain-soaked reality that the dead person isn't returning. But unlike loved ones who die physically, our dead self returns in some part as we treat our neurons and work out our grief consciously and subconsciously. Eventually, my counterfactual thinking about the crash faded from my mind.

Book Reading Regret

Books accompanied me wherever I went. Novels enticed me to read them at home over lunch, at break time, when I could make time. Non-fiction satiated my curiosity about anything, or taught me how to market the books I wanted to write. I would've happily read anything, anytime, anywhere; but some weren't so happy about my voracious reading. My ex preferred me to watch TV with him, not read a book beside him. He wasn't a reader; he grew up in houses barren with books. Perhaps that's why he complained I read too much. But he wasn't the first to say so. I'd heard that refrain since grade 5. I attempted to read less and restricted my mass paperback novel habit to three per week.

I wish I hadn't.

don't restrict what you love doing to make others happy →

Catastrophic injury crystallizes the choices we made. Those we made to keep loved ones, peers, societal expectations happy glare regret like a sun flare off a mirror. What was the harm of me reading as many novels as I wanted when I read them while alone? Why was me reading and him watching TV so bad when we're sharing the couch? Why was reading characterized as a waste of time when television or running or truncating sleep for the sake of more work wasn't? It's strange what others think we should do with our time, yet don't want us to have any say in what they do with theirs.

For me, reading was stress relief. But, more importantly, reading is the number one advice famous authors give to burgeoning writers. Reading is part of what I do and who I am. I regret allowing others to turn it into a sin and deciding for me how much I should read.

Who could ever imagine I'd lose my ability to read? What seemed like no big deal to make others happy became a big deal when I lost my reading comprehension for 18 years. As the years droned on, reading loss metastasized into gargantuan grief because of all the books I hadn't read and a future devoid of them. Regret clawed at me. I wrote books, blogs, and *Psychology Today* posts on reading to unhook regret's talons from my flesh, but only Lindamood-Bell restoring my reading comprehension, freed me.

What do you regret most? What counterfactual thinking is eating up your brain space? Let's start on the next Action Plan.

LEARN MORE

You can read more about reading loss and regaining reading comprehension in my memoir and *Psychology Today* posts at https://www.psychologytoday.com/blog/concussion-is-brain-injury.

Action Plan: What Will You Do Differently When You Heal?

After deep breathing for a couple of minutes and setting up your reward and stress buster for completing this step, turn to a fresh page in your *Stress and Grieving* notebook and title it "Regrets."

What Do You Regret?

Write freely all you regret. You may have only one regret or dozens.

From your list, choose the regret that drumbeats in your mind and erupts tears in the night's deepest hours.

Name that regret and write it as a heading.

Then write the story of that regret. Take stock of your choices and why you made them. And identify if your regret is counterfactual thinking about the circumstances that lead to your brain injury.

Counter Your Regret

Now write the heading "What I Will Do Differently."

Like with my reading loss for the 18 years after the 2000 car crash, you may not have an opportunity to do different. But before you can act differently, you have to think differently. Good thoughts lead to good words, which lead to good action.

Rewrite the story with what you'd do differently.

Ask yourself if you really would choose differently or if you'd fall back into the same decisions you made pre-injury because you want to make people happy or the choices are so engrained. Be honest. There's no one around to judge you or whom you need to impress. It's just you.

For me, the message that reading is a time waster, of no use, was so engrained that today the idea of reading whenever I want—under the limitations of my energy and cognitive ability—still creates guilt. Countering this reaction becomes a therapeutic dose—a cognitive-behavioural therapy moment—where I remind myself that reading is necessary for writing, for my peace of mind, and for my physical health. I remind myself and my neurodoc that brain biofeedback shows clearly that my brainwaves and heart rate improve when I read. Anything that improves brain function and lowers stress markers, which reading does for me, is vital.

Changing Engrained Thought Patterns

What can you do to prevent yourself from falling back into old habits, staying in regret? Is there a mantra or routine that could counter that falling back?

List what will help you think differently so that you don't repeat any of your regrets. Include small but significant rewards or accountability methods. The latter may be possible if you have a supportive person or therapist in your life as vested as you are to heal that regret.

You may never be able to do things differently. But if you gain that opportunity, you've prepared yourself to make different choices and to succeed so that you don't repeat your regrets.

Repeat this Action Plan for each of your important regrets that affected your life in ways you'd like to change.

For counterfactual thinking, list the facts that belie this false thinking. Remember that what happened, happened. You cannot change the past.

Forgive Yourself

And lastly, forgive yourself. (Return to the Forgiveness section in Step Two if you need to.) Tell yourself you made the best choices you could at the time. Your brain injury has given you the radical opportunity to see the choice for what it was, to learn from it, and to live differently. See also Step Four, Healing Grief.

CHAPTER 21

TRAUMA

Pre-Injury Wounds and Traumas Reanimate

Like happened with me, your brain injury may have disconnected your pre-injury memories from your emotions, and thus undone any trauma work you may have done back before your injury. When emotions return, the now unhealed memories upthrust a tsunami of traumas that we hadn't thought about in years. They lash against our mind, making us feel out of time. Confusion piles on top of flashbacks, and chaos results.

Acknowledge Traumas Being Unhealed

To re-heal these pre-injury wounds, you and your therapist will need to acknowledge this strange unhealing and work together to reconnect the memories with the emotions. Strategies, medications, and rest will not restore your affect so that you can do this work. Only neurostimulation therapies can. (See Step Five for treating your neurons, including your emotions.) When those broken memory-emotion neural networks reconnect, we embark on a chaotic road towards unifying memory and emotion, one that requires cognitive empathy from the therapist and perseverance and courage from us.

> *cognitive empathy is the health care professional putting themself in our shoes and responding to our distress with kindness* →

Our memories appearing and disappearing like whack-a-mole or black holes opening and closing in our memory banks complicate trying to re-heal pre-injury traumas. Although neurostimulation therapies may regenerate the regions responsible for long-term autobiographical memory, working through grief may become necessary before trauma memories stabilize enough to reconnect to emotions. Grieving may do that work without us realizing it.

> *neurostimulation, cognitive empathy, and grief work stabilize the memory-emotion disconnect* →

I found that this trauma unhealing is not discussed during neuro-rehab. A decade passed before my neurodoc identified it. My gamma brainwave enhancement training brought this issue to the fore. Guiding me to reconnect my memories to their emotional resolution would've been pioneering, but unfortunately my neurodoc didn't pursue it with me, and I discovered you can't really do it on your own. Some healing work requires another person, a person willing to learn, listen compassionately, and guide you towards this goal. I manage the lack of such a person in my life through some of the work I outline in Step Four.

LEARN MORE

> For more on cognitive empathy, see https://www.psychologytoday.com/ca/blog/concussion-is-brain-injury/201805/cognitive-empathy-reading-loss-after-brain-injury.
>
> And for a discussion on health care professionals partnering with patients in their healing, see https://www.psychologytoday.com/ca/blog/concussion-is-brain-injury/201907/why-doctors-must-listen-people-brain-injury.

Trauma After Injury

After the injury, come the social traumas. Rejections, judgements, labelling, and exploitation. Those tasked to heal, the neurologists and psychiatrists, present their methods as the most up-to-date yet leave you struggling with brain injury's catastrophic cognitive, emotional, and metabolic effects. Their abandonment traumatizes.

being alone creates its own continuing trauma →

I believe these three sources of trauma worsen brain injury and exacerbate dysfunction.

Trauma's psychic pain knifes every cell and bleeds into every facet of life.

Fiction Depicts Trauma's Distorting Death Grip

Jean-Guy Beauvoir is a fictional character in Louise Penny's Chief Inspector Gamache mystery series. He's a thirty-something Inspector in the Sûreté du Québec, once married, loyal to his boss, Armand Gamache, shot in the line of duty, and addicted to OxyContin. Through Beauvoir, we descend into psychic pain; his trauma creates paranoia and rage, making him exploitable for nefarious ends. The evil character in *How The Lights Gets In* uses him to find and eradicate Gamache.

> "Beauvoir hadn't asked why they wanted to go to Three Pines, or why the unmarked Sûreté van was following them.
>
> He didn't care.
>
> He was just a chauffeur. He'd do as he was told. No more debate. He'd learned that when he cared, he got hurt, and he couldn't take any more pain. Even the pills couldn't dull it anymore."

Even though Beauvoir experienced trauma without brain injury, Penny aptly describes the emotional state we share with him. But how many endeavour to imagine being in psychic pain while living with unhealed brain injury and floundering to live up to people's expectations to be functional? It's impossible!

Medication Isn't Enough

At some point, psychic pain after brain injury and abandonment becomes so vast and entrenched that medication cannot address it.

Primitive Trauma Therapy

One day, I asked my neurodoc about trauma therapy. He said, "It's primitive." Despite all the work into post-traumatic stress disorder (PTSD), he admitted what I'd experienced with him and with my other brain injury specialists: PTSD therapy is a work in progress that doesn't live up to its hype. "You too can get better!" we each discover independently isn't really true, and we wonder if it's just us. It isn't.

 I think one enormous obstacle is that we don't actually know what trauma does to the brain. We're learning about the role of microglia, about how early trauma changes the way we see the world, about using therapeutic doses to treat that kind of trauma. But how does continuing trauma of forced aloneness complicate brain injury? Is it its own kind of brain injury?

 Forced isolation destroys trust; social skills atrophy. Without trust, we cannot create or maintain healthy relationships.

 Brain injury already interferes with that process through damage to concentration, memory, communication abilities, and so on. Those losses create another kind of mistrust: mistrusting our own ability to understand social interactions, to sense who's trustworthy and who's not, and to express what we're thinking.

 Learning that people can endanger healing combined with mistrusting our ability to know who to trust closes us down. We avoid talking about our grief; we become alert to accusations of thinking negatively or signs of boredom or rolling eyes or finding an excuse to change the subject or hearing, "There you go again. Can't you talk about anything else?"

 I believe trauma fundamentally arises from broken bonds between loved ones or trusted professionals and their clients.

Protecting Ourself

I'm one of those small percentage of people for whom morphine doesn't work to dull pain. Since medication for physical pain was out, I searched for alternatives and found remedies for psychic pain.

But I believe the best trauma therapy centres on creating experiences with humans that strengthen bonds, create trust, and support and encourage. We begin with one person, meeting them regularly and frequently, under the guidance of an experienced therapist. When we build trust with them, it counters the conditioning that trust is impossible. This relationship becomes a model for rebuilding trust with others. But finding that is like navigating in pitch black with glimpses of light. Whenever I found support, the person became seriously ill, moved away, was available for a limited time, or, in the case of health care professionals, not quite as advertised.

The corollary to creating this kind of experience is separating from those people who caused harm and are unrepentant. Like encasing a broken leg in a cast then continuing to smack it, you can't heal an injury if it keeps being assaulted. Separation frees up energy to focus on functionality, treating the neurons, and discovering what gives meaning in life. This kind of work restores trust in ourself.

NEVERENDING *grief*
Neverending **HEALING**

Step Four

HEALING GRIEF

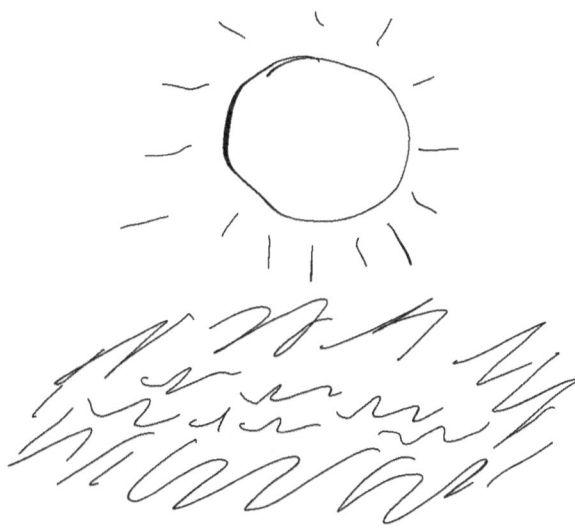

CHAPTER 22

YOU ARE NOT THE INJURY

A reminder that you are not the injury. Review your injury newsletter in your *Stress and Grieving* notebook and compare it to your strengths and Optimism Test results. Notice how your cognitive challenges differ from your strengths and talents, the aspects of you. Brain injury-caused challenges impede expressing who you are, but your injury is not you.

To be honest, I don't know if healing neurons must come before healing brain injury grief or if vice versa is best. But I know that treating neurons and healing grief can co-occur. If you're ready to dive into diagnosing what's happening in your brain and treating your neurons effectively, go to Step Five. Once you start that process, return here to continue this one. Without healing grief, treating your neurons only gets you so far before the grief drags your recovery backwards.

Action Plan: You Are What God or the Cosmos Says You Are

Humans don't decide who you are. God created you. Nature formed you out of the light and energy of the cosmos. Those creating forces set you on the path of who you are.

Bad things happened to you. Really bad. Perhaps like me, fear and anxiety dog your steps every moment.

Opportunities to heal turn to dust as we walk down the promised road. The proverbial door shuts, but we feel a breeze, turn, and see an open window. As we climb out, the upper sash slams down on our back. Why do we try so hard when delays, obstacles, good things keep turning to bad? A dog in the park saunters over to snuffle hello and demand attention. Stroking the soft dog fur, a surge of energy refills us with tangible hope. With such moments, we take two steps forward and believe, guardedly perhaps, that now we'll be able to return to work, as standard medical care had promised. Then neuro-fatigue descends like the sky crashing to earth, smothering us, and we slide backwards in our exercise goals and work opportunities.

Hope vanishes into a tiny cockroach crack. And the couch and TV become our best friends.

Since you're reading this book, hope glimmers still in your heart, despite standard brain injury care not assessing your brain activity properly, not treating you with neurostimulation, and your social support limps along or is gone. By reading this book, you're shouting at the unkind world that you're still trying and all the steps backwards don't decide how your story ends. Your brain injury may show a false face to the world of who you are, but it and what people say about you don't decide who you really are.

Brain injury and learnt mistrust distort how we express ourself, impede us being us, but as I talked about in Step One, we are a loved creation. Yet it's one thing to know, it's another to act that knowledge out. I struggle with giving up, quitting, letting the delays and obstacles and stream of challenges without end halt my steps forward. And then something gets me up in the morning. I try again. No matter how much I don't want to try again, how much I want to tuck my head in and stay where it's safe, I comply with the creative, loving force that gets me up to read or write or walk or make that phone call that overwhelms me. When I'm up, I can take that one step that leads to the next and the next. Then rest for a while.

Persistence and rest work together to keep us from stagnating in brain injury. Brain injury creates a seven times increased risk of developing dementia. Although we don't know if neurostimulation reduces that risk, we're already seeing it helps slow or stop Alzheimer's. That, alone, leads to the reasonable assumption that neurostimulation will decrease our risk closer to normal. When we understand that and know a larger force cares for us, then taking the next step becomes doable in our minds. Remembering that God loves you—that you're an integral part of the cosmos—helps to counter despair. I hope this book may give you courage to grab effective neurostimulation and neuromodulation treatments for your brain despite all the naysayers and obstacles.

Your Personal Reminder

Rest your eyes on the words and image you pinned up as part of Action Plan: Contemplate Being Loved in Step One. Feel their love and comfort soak into you. Do this whenever your hope flags.

Action Plan: Bibliotherapy or Movie Therapy

Bibliotherapy is a new, growing form of therapy. After I regained my reading comprehension, I inadvertently fell into using it to heal my grief. It can complement neurostimulation and neuromodulation therapies after your neurons have begun to reboot, repair, and rewire. See Step Five: Treating Your Neurons for more.

I think readers naturally find therapy in novels. Attending a clinic that uses Lindamood-Bell's visualizing and verbalizing program to restore reading comprehension is essential to benefit from bibliotherapy. However, movie therapy can work in the absence of restored reading comprehension. Usually health care professionals trained in bibliotherapy conduct it. But we can do it for ourself and use Mind Alive's SMR for Reading audiovisual entrainment protocol prior to or during bibliotherapy.

Choose a Novel That Talks About What You're Struggling With

Basically, bibliotherapy involves choosing a novel that explores the issues you need therapy for or you're grieving. Sometimes, you may find you're experiencing bibliotherapy inadvertently as you read a favourite author and realize their characters are struggling with the same problems as you are. Reading these characters' journeys unearths emotions, thoughts, and grief and will help you come to grips with your brain injury and how it radically altered your life. Seeing how fictional characters cope with similar feelings helps you cope.

LEARN MORE

> "Restoring reading comprehension means just that: once again being able to comprehend articles and books that you want to or need to read. It doesn't mean using strategies to simulate reading. It means restored reading." Bibliotherapy is best done after you've undergone proper

assessment of your reading comprehension and had visualizing and verbalizing retraining. See https://concussionisbraininjury.com/treatments/visualizing-and-verbalizing-restoring-reading-comprehension/.

Movie Therapy

You may find movie therapy a suitable alternative and easier. Sometimes, we need a funny movie to lift our mood, to help us escape our daily struggles. Animations don't strain the brain and are fun. Make watching comedies and animations a habit as part of your stress-relieving activities.

When you're struggling with grief or a stressful situation, a movie in which characters are wrestling with similar issues may help you understand your own better. Such a movie may also give you ideas on how to cope or make you feel less alone.

Another form of movie therapy is to choose a TV series that focuses on the goodness of humans, like *Star Trek*. This series and its spin-offs mostly view the future as a good place in which humans wrestle with grief and the same situations we face and come together to heal and solve problems. The characters' teamwork may make you pine for what you don't have, but imagining something better instead of dystopian futures can stoke your hope. It's important to support and empower your hope. When we're alone in our brain injury, hope falters or dies. So anything that can fuel it keeps us going.

The Work

Settle into your quiet place with your chosen bibliotherapy book. Have a notebook or tablet with you while you're reading.

When you read a scene or dialogue that resonates with your own struggles or injury, stop reading. Reread it. Perhaps bookmark the page and highlight or underline the passage that sticks out in your mind. Allow the words to sink into your mind. Jot down in your notebook your thoughts and emotions as you process those resonating words in the novel. If the scene brings up a repeating theme in your life, you'll want to talk it over with your therapist. To remember to do that, open your calendar and edit your therapy appointment by adding notes on this theme, how the novel presented it, and any thoughts it brought up. **Remember**: ask your therapist to ask you to check your calendar appointment notes to guard against forgetting.

If you don't have a therapist, perhaps talk to your local Help line about it or trusted clergy. Have your notebook handy so that when you call the Help line, you'll be able to refer to it to remember your thoughts and feelings the novel brought up.

When you've taken the time to process that scene or dialogue, continue to read.

Follow the same procedure for movie therapy.

If you have a short attention span and scattered memory, watch the entire movie first to gain a sense of what it's about, then re-watch it at a later date and follow the above procedure for movie therapy.

A Few Words on Grieving

A few years ago, I watched a show that followed a family group of elephants. This noisy family group came across a corpse. The bones lay on the dusty path. I didn't recognize the remains as an elephant. But the group did. They stopped. They gathered a little way around the corpse as they quieted. One stepped forward and stretched her trunk to smell them. She flattened the end of her trunk on a bone to inhale every scent molecule left. As the others drew closer, she raised her left forefoot and swung it like a metronome towards the skull without touching it. The family rumbled deep in their throats, a backdrop of rising volume, then quiet, then rising again. Rumbling vibrates the ground, sending messages to any elephant that can hear. The group, one by one, grasped small bones, lifted the skull, held tiny, thin bones in their mouths, cradled them in their trunks. The elephants fell silent as they paid homage to and held close the long-dead elephant. After a few minutes, they carried on their way, enthusiastically greeting another elephant family.

LEARN MORE

Find the clip of the elephants mourning the dead on BBC Studios YouTube channel at https://youtu.be/C5RiHT-SXK2A

Grief, Human Style

Grief follows a kind of pattern. We learn about the death. We reach out to the dead person's family and talk to mutual friends to process and understand it. We respect the mourners and care for them, bringing them food and listening as they weep and talk. We pull out old photographs to showcase at the funeral and watch the funeral parlour's slideshow. We write on social media what's happened, maybe blog about the dead person whom we miss terribly. We write eulogies and read them to the mourners at memorials and funerals. Afterwards, we gather to celebrate and reminisce about the dead person's life. We pay homage to the dead person and cradle the mourning. Then we call it time and leave. But unlike ancient cultures who held longer mourning periods, our modern society cuts the grieving process short. And since brain injury grief is pretty much unrecognized, we don't get a chance to grieve our own death through injury at all.

Therapy Doesn't Include Grieving Brain Injury

A few brain injury specialists may consider helping us grieve our death through brain injury. But mostly we're on our own. On top of that, we're alone. Isolation traumatizes daily. It's like being in solitary, with no exit possible. But unlike solitary in a prison where an inhuman justice system pays guards to isolate the convicted, isolation in the community arises from loved ones unloving us, breaking their promise to support and be there, no matter what.

Traditionally, grieving is a community event—even in modern times where busy-ness trumps community gathering, where we restrict funeral parlour visitations and set timelines on memorials. Westerners squirm when death sidles close; they hop in and out of funerals like birds flitting away from cats. They avoid obvious death, use euphemisms to throw blankets over it, and refuse to countenance the idea that brain injury killed us and we're living in this hell of being dead while being very much alive. Most don't acknowledge we need to mourn our own passing, to heal our continuing trauma of forced aloneness.

How can we get better when brain injury grief isn't addressed, when psychic pain is allowed to spread, when trauma continues daily under the burden of isolation? The fictional character Beauvoir speaks the truth: after a while, pills cannot dull the pain. Medication is not the answer.

Understanding Is Part of Grieving

Understanding is part of grieving. In the previous sections, we excavated our grief. But we need to do more than face our grief. We need to mourn and heal.

We talk to understand what we're grieving, and we talk to mourn and heal. A variety of cultural rituals around grieving extend beyond talking. So how do we grieve without community in our aloneness? How do we learn who's safe to talk to? How does continuing trauma affect our grieving?

How Do We Grieve Our Brain Injury?

Grieving isn't a onetime thing nor a 12-week cognitive-behavioural-therapy program. Although grieving diminishes over time, it returns unexpectedly. Like the elephants showed when they happened unexpectedly upon the bones on their path, whenever we come across remnants of our dead self, don't resist the upwelling grief. Stop to respect, cry, and hold our old self in love. Then after a few minutes, carry on our way. Perhaps we can follow the elephants' example while also borrowing from our traditional ways of grieving. Let's pay homage to and cradle our dead self in order to say goodbye.

CHAPTER 23

ACTION PLAN: SAYING AU REVOIR TO YOU

Talking About It

"One day, Glenda had gently spoken to me about positive talk. She related that it was amazing how the corporate environment changed when people were banned from making negative statements. I listened, straining my brain to grasp what she was saying, to absorb her point that my talk was negative: the pain, the fatigue, my husband leaving, feeling unable to cope with taking on a tenant like he wanted me to, the insurance company denying another treatment plan, and the rehab homework and my hopes for it working. Her words echoed what others had said. My brain injury and seatbelt injuries had eaten up my life. There was no room for work. Energy drained out of my cheeks, and my body grew heavy as I struggled to shut my mouth against mentioning to her whatever sensation or thought or errant feeling popped into my consciousness to comply with what they all wanted to hear.

Action Plan: Saying Au Revoir to You

It was a losing battle. I needed to talk out what I didn't understand. And I didn't understand this injury of the brain."

From Concussion Is Brain Injury: Treating the Neurons and Me.

Journalling

If you're not journalling yet, begin. Find a lined journal you like. Purchase a bunch of them from a bulk buy store with lots of pens that write easily. When you have little energy, a pen that flows ink smoothly on a page lets you write a little longer.

Whenever you journal, write the date first. It grounds you in the present. Seeing the dates helps you see your progress. Write about the loss, your old self, the things you miss, whatever appears on the page. I used to limit myself to pleasant events because facing the bad overwhelmed me and because messages of gratitude and positive thinking spill out from the TV, newspapers, articles, and people's mouths. But it isn't positive to cover over the pain.

gratitude isn't truth when it's used to stuff down grief →

Journalling starts the process of grieving and understanding. Talking bolsters it through mithra and by using another communication form, the oral form.

But who to talk to when we're alone or our brain injury therapist wants us to focus on the positive? Does anyone tell a grieving parent to see the positive side of losing their child?!

I talked a lot about the car crash that destroyed my life until my family and friends wanted me to shut up already. Insurance companies and various specialists, though, forced me to talk over and over about the crash to gather information on me, to find reasons to reject my claim, or simply to take a history. By the time we settled my insurance battles, I didn't want to talk about the crash anymore. I no longer associated talking with healing, with understanding my brain injury and processing the grief, but with my words being used against me. I continue to work on unlearning that.

Blogging

A social worker suggested I blog about my brain injury because I'd been barred from expressing myself for years. That began the grieving process. Yet I still had to find a trustable therapist who'd listen for as long as I needed to talk, no matter how much I meandered before what was bothering me poured out. I needed a listener who'd refrain from telling me to see the positive side of losing myself. There's a difference between discovering gifts after brain injury versus being told to see the loss as positive. The former enhances awareness of your altered self; the latter stops the grieving process and stagnates healing.

Talking

If you have a trustworthy therapist who'll let you meander in your telling without interrupting you or countering with, "One positive thing is...," set up a therapy goal of grieving your brain injury and your lost self using therapeutic doses. Therapeutic doses will allow you to meander into and out of painful moments, moments and experiences you've stuffed down for years. You may talk about your grief for a few seconds or minutes in a session before rambling to something else. But keep at it over months and years, making it a regular part of therapy. This is a long process, not a short-term fix. You'll know it's helping when you don't instantly become numb or sob as you relate some part of the event or the self you lost.

Help lines help!

If you don't have a therapist, call your local Help Line. Call, don't text unless you're mute or non-verbal. Verbal communication complements journalling, no matter how difficult your brain injury, trauma, and grief makes speaking your thoughts.

Remember: when a person dies, we first talk about the event and them. Help lines receive regular callers, not only ones in immediate distress. Don't be shy. Call. They won't judge you for calling, even nightly, to talk out your grief.

Journalling After Talking

Write in your journal any thoughts and feelings that come up during the talking session to assist processing and talking's healing effects. Write about the scenes you talked about or refer to them in shorthand; perhaps describe how the person you were talking to reacted. Sometimes we see what's not there; putting it down in black-and-white helps us reflect on our perceptions.

Depending on the frequency of therapy, you may need to journal for several days on the session to continue processing the thoughts that came up or record related memories that appeared in the succeeding days. Reflect on why those memories emerged. How do you feel? What grief did your talking and journalling unearth that you want to explore in the next session or Help Line talk? Write that unearthed emotion and related memories not only in the journal but also in your calendar for the next session to hopefully remind you at the time of your appointment. I say hopefully because we can forget to look at our notes. Consider asking your therapist to have you check if you've written any notes for that day's session, to protect against forgetting.

Talk to Your Pre-Injury Self

We've all had moments of talking out loud to ourself. We berate or instruct ourself on how to pour the right amount of milk into our cereal. Or we remonstrate ourself not to be late. For this exercise, let's talk to our pre-injury self. Not berate or instruct or remind, but express our thoughts and feelings, ask questions, and listen.

Set up your usual rewards and stress busters, then find a safe place where you can lie down on the ground, or as close to the Earth as possible, undisturbed by people or animals. If you don't like bugs and have access to a clean basement, lying down on a basement floor poured right over the ground works, too. A rug or yoga mat may soften its hardness. Or if you can't do either, lie down on the floor closest to the ground. Deep breathe for a few minutes, stretching your senses mentally to feel the Earth's harmonics.

Our planet has an electromagnetic field vibrating at 7.83 Hz, which is called the "Schumann resonance" named after Dr. Winfried O. Schumann who mathematically predicted it in 1952. Theta brainwaves are in the meditative range of 7 to 8 Hz—the twilight zone where our minds wander, not asleep yet not fully engaged with the day.

Our planet Earth supports us and heals us

Lying on the ground in a safe space will prime your mind for imagining your pre-injury self and starting a conversation with them. Start talking out loud to your pre-injury self when you're ready.

If you're at risk of choking when talking flat on your back, sit up. Lean against a tree if you can, for trees de-stress us while we sit on the ground, still in contact with our planet Earth.

Express, Ask, and Listen

Imagine you're facing your pre-injury self. Speak to them your thoughts and feelings, whatever comes to mind. Imagine your pre-injury self listening. Pause now and then to listen to their replies. Perhaps they will exhume a memory relating to your thoughts or evoking similar feelings. If counterfactual thinking around your brain injury consumes your energy—or you feel guilty you brought it on—speak out loud those shame-filled thoughts, the fateful decisions you made. Hear your pre-injury self neutralize your counterfactual thinking, explain why they did what they did. Ask questions that have been lingering in your subconscious. Listen to their answers, and feel their love for you.

Tell them you welcome parts of them to return to you when you heal your brain. Express which parts you most want back and why. Ask your pre-injury self if they're ready to be reborn and merge with who you are now, leaving behind the worst and bringing with them the best of who they were. Listen to their answer; assure them you're OK with the parts you yearn for not being exactly the same as before.

Healing Old Self-Loathing

If self-loathing formed part of your former pre-injury self, address that from your current perspective. Read out loud Step One sections on mithra and love, and proclaim they, too, were loved and interconnected with all of humanity. Listen or intuitively feel their response. This process will take time. See the next section for more on healing self-loathing.

Therapeutic Dosing

Do this exercise in therapeutic doses that you can handle. It may only be ten seconds or an hour several times a week. Or maybe 15 minutes once a month. Whatever you can handle, time is irrelevant. It's not about some standard to measure up to or what a clinic allows. It's about what works for you to say au revoir to your pre-injury self and make peace with the decisions you made that lead to your brain injury and to your regrets.

After a therapeutic dose, slowly return to your regular world. Don't rush it. Like with using audiovisual entrainment for calming or meditating, transitioning from this kind of introspective state is less of a shock when you do it unhurriedly. And don't forget to reward yourself when done!

Cradle Yourself

Grief makes us feel that all there is is pain and a bleak future. Burying the grief hardens your heart into a rock filled with the gunpowder of rage and depression. But cradling yourself in these moments lets the feelings out, the thoughts know they're OK, and you to heal one therapeutic dose at a time.

One devastating day, amid hard years, my pastor recommended I collect "good girl" instances and put them in a folder to look at when life overwhelms me.

cradle yourself with your good-person folder ➤

The idea is simple: print out social media comments, emails and messages, kudos, any awards, NaNoWriMo winner certificates or other kinds of certificates, and such like that reflect how people see you as a good person and/or are physical evidence of your achievements. Collect writings that say what people like about you, times people helped you, times you helped others, your achievements, no matter how small you or others may regard them. Collect the same in paper form. For example, when you're mentioned in books or articles or if anyone has used you as a character in a novel or short story, newsletters that mention you or you wrote for, letters to the editor or politicians when you objected to their mithra-destroying policies.

Gather these printouts and clippings into a folder and label it "Good__" and fill in your name. Place the folder where you can easily see it so you don't forget you have it or where it is. Open it to look through when despair grips you and hope has fled. Let these writings remind you that others think you're a good person, that people like you, and that you've done good things and achieved goals, including the smallest ones like making oatmeal. Every small goal met is one step forward.

don't discount the smallest of achievements →

If you have degrees or college certificates or continuing education certificates that you haven't framed, frame them and hang them up where they face you when you're on the computer.

Even though I earned my Bachelor of Science degree decades ago when my brain was firing on all cylinders and today I cannot imagine being able to do that, my degree hangs above my computer facing me where I cannot forget nor discount it. My ex and a friend had it framed back when I was in my twenties (before my brain injury) and needed to see my degree for what it was: a significant achievement.

A Quiet Space

If you haven't yet created a quiet space for reading this book or resting with a cup of coffee or tea, do it now. It doesn't have to be big.

My spiritual mentor had a small table set against one wall of her yellow-painted office. Two small stuffed chairs faced each other next to the table. Hers faced the window, the one I sat in faced the closed door and a wall poster of flowers. A small lamp, items that had spiritual value to her, and a candle graced the table. She'd light the candle when we sat down and blow it out when our time was done. She advised me to create a space for myself where I could sit quietly, reflect, or prepare for the day.

A quiet space was the antithesis of how I was brought up and one more unwelcome lifestyle change brought on by my brain injury. But I felt cradled in her quiet space and wanted the same for myself.

there is no failure in taking years to set up a quiet space for yourself →

I spent years pondering, hemming and hawing, before deciding where and how to set up my quiet space. Mine ended up being a large, comfy chair with a footstool and cushions at my back, next to a window and a small table in my kitchen. I don't have a candle, though I have many candles, usually unlit, in various places. I'd like to have a candle I can light safely when I sit to read. And perhaps, one day, I'll figure out how to make that happen.

Action Plan: Saying Au Revoir to You

your quiet space can evolve over the years as you heal

Your quiet space can be in a small room or part of a large space. You can start with just a chair and add to it over weeks, months, or years. If you're living with other people, ensure they know and respect that this is *your* quiet space.

If you live with people who don't give a damn and will fill it up with clutter and use it for themselves, then perhaps find a place outdoors you can go to. Someone once told me they had a favourite bench near a river in downtown Toronto, where they sat to talk to Jesus. They sit quietly there when others are unlikely to disturb them.

Don't eat in your quiet space. You want the space to nourish you. Emotional eating will have the opposite effect. Maybe have a glass of water, sparkling or plain, or a cup of coffee or tea without milk, cream, or sugar, something low calorie but no diet drinks since artificial sweeteners can affect brain function and your weight opposite to what you want.

LEARN MORE

If you put a lot of milk, cream, and/or sugar in your coffee or tea, reduce the sugar first a little at a time every day. Your tastebuds will habituate until you no longer like it with sugar. Repeat with the milk or cream until you have your tea or coffee black. You'll find that you'll seek good quality tea and coffee, and your tastebuds will notice the taste differences between roasts and varietals. This is good for your brain, relearning to distinguish between different tastes. Even better, you can use an **occasional** latte or cappuccino as a treat, since milk in your coffee will no longer be the norm. Do something similar with hot chocolate. Make it with dark chocolate mix and use skim or 1% milk. Then, as a **rare** reward treat, add extra chocolate or a small scoop of ice cream.

When brain injury distorts taste, choose better quality lemon curd, organic jam, or chocolate because they have stronger flavour notes that don't rely on sugar and salt. Because it costs more, you'll eat less. Because you eat less, you savour it in order to extend it. Chewing slowly, taking small bites turns eating into a mindful moment. The present moment becomes a moment of pleasure.

Nature, a Place to Feel Loved

Trees nurture. They instill calm. Flowers delight us with their beauty. Birds amuse, and squirrels make us grin. Find a place and time where you can enjoy the natural world as often as possible. Daily is best. But even if it's a once weekly slow shuffle to a struggling tree in a ragged park, that tree and that walk can still bring peace into your mind.

When I visited Milan decades ago, I noticed a lack of parks. Toronto has so much greenery that walking amongst beautiful architecture in that Italian city with nary a tree in sight felt alien. Then I spotted a small bumpy area of green. Neglected, forlorn, the grass and suffering trees still lifted my spirit. They reconnected me to the world I knew.

Walk in a park or ravine or wood however long you can when you can. And if your energy is low, simply sit on your steps, your balcony, or porch and let your gaze fall on the trees, sky, clouds, water, grass, flowers or dormant bushes; listen to the birds and watch the antics of passing dogs, squirrels, chipmunks, or your local fauna; write poetry in your smart phone; snap photos even if they'll remain unlooked at.

taking photos allows you to really see what's caught your eye

Sometimes you may want to take a quick shot; other times, take longer to frame it, to figure out what is the most important thing you want in your photo.

Watch people as they pass by and make up stories about them in your head. Brain injury affects imagination, yet trying to spend a few seconds on creating stories about passersby helps to take you out of your own life and slowly, slowly teaches your brain a new skill.

Cradling yourself is not a linear behaviour, but one you insert regularly into your day. In small moments like enjoying every morsel of your favourite bread or big like hugging a tree, cradling nourishes and unwinds you in between grief work and after therapy, doctors' appointments, and difficult personal interactions.

Action Plan: Saying Au Revoir to You

Collect Photos and Stories of Yourself

Photos, videos, and albums are the visual story of your pre-injury self and life and document the post-injury you. Just as we spend time together poring over photos of deceased family, sharing stories those photos bring up, so, too, you can spend time with your photos, remembering the stories of who you were. Spending that time, here and there, in moments or hours, in therapeutic doses, facilitates mourning. When you close the album or turn off the digital frame for the last time, you'll feel more ready to say goodbye to your pre-injury self.

Physical Photos and Albums

Depending on your age, you may or may not have stacks of photos in boxes or physical albums. First, gather them together and choose an easily recalled storage area where you can find them quickly. Second, find an empty box or spare album and label it "Grieving." Use this box to place photos in that you find hard to look at and need to mourn later.

You may need to spend several sessions of five minutes here, five minutes there when you have the energy to find all your physical photos and albums to put them in the accessible storage area.

Digital Photos

Create an album on your phone, tablet, or computer labelled "Grieving." File the digital photos in there that bring up painful, grieving memories.

Mourning Through Photos

Once you've organized your photos, sit in your quiet space and randomly peruse the photos or flip through the albums. This part of the Action Plan is about grieving memories in therapeutic doses when you have the sudden urge to spend a few minutes with your memories or when a memory pops into your head and you want to find its visual record to help you remember and mourn it.

Stories

Use these times with your photos and albums to drive your journalling. In your journal, write your feelings, thoughts, and memories that came up as you looked at your photos that day. Seeing the photos may create one emotion while the memories bring back different emotions of that time. Record both emotions.

writing a story of a photo helps to process the memory and reconnect it to your emotions
———————▶

In your *Stress and Grieving* notebook, use the photos to spur you into writing the story that runs round in your head. You don't need to journal memories that bring only peace or happiness or when it's so painful, you can't at this point in time think about them. But if you feel grief or feel the need to work something out about it, then writing the story will help you process and work it out.

If you find yourself stuck because of fragmented memories or the pain is too great, try writing a fictional story starring your pre-injury self. This can take the form of a short story, a comic strip, a graphic novel, poetry, or whatever form best suits your ability. Sign up for the free global National Novel Writing Month (NaNoWriMo); use their resources as external Go buttons to initiate you to write your stories.

when your Go button—your ability to initiate—is off, external resources can push it on
———————▶

You don't have to write a novel during November's NaNoWriMo nor do you have to write only in November. You can write whatever you want, at any time, and track your personal goal(s) on the NaNoWriMo website. Your goals can comprise words, pages, hours, or whatever. Their resources will help you track your progress; their pep talks will soften your aloneness. As you know from occupational therapy, seeing your progress is like receiving a gold star when you were a kid. A reward and a reminder you're getting there.

Action Plan: Saying Au Revoir to You

Write an Eulogy

After you've spent time with your photos, journalled your thoughts and emotions, written stories about what you grieve most intensely or frequently, it's time to write a eulogy about your pre-injury self. A eulogy comprises praise, funny stories, heartwarming moments, and what you miss about the dead.

web pages galore teach how to write a eulogy

Various websites teach different approaches to writing a eulogy. Find one that appeals to you. Print out the instructions and slip it into your *Stress and Grieving* notebook. Slip in with the instructions photo prints that particularly speak to you. Or create a new digital album and label it "Eulogy."

When you're ready to start, sit in your quiet space, spend a couple of minutes deep breathing, decide on your reward for starting or continuing your eulogy, and have your stress busters ready.

1. Take out the eulogy-writing instructions and related photos.
2. Start writing.
3. *Remember*: there is no rush as your eulogy has no funeral-mandated deadline. You may have only enough physical energy to write for 10 minutes or emotional energy for five minutes. Even one minute is better than no minutes.
4. Repeat the preparation instructions each time you sit down to work on your eulogy. Although you began working on your eulogy in your quiet space, you may want to continue it at your computer, where you can type it up easier. Or you may prefer to handwrite it on a notepad or a new paperblanks journal. Attach photos where appropriate or wait until you're fully finished before attaching them. Perhaps draw or doodle in places to further express what you're feeling or thinking about your lost self.
5. Add to your eulogy your pre-injury self's favourite music. Perhaps play these songs as you're writing. Or if you're like me and can't listen to music and write at the same time, listen to them and lose yourself in them before working on your eulogy. You may find yourself crying for quite a while, so it's good if you do this in a private place where you won't be disturbed. You need to be free to

grieve without people interrupting you with their judgements or demands to get on with chores or life.

Writing your eulogy may take months or a year or an hour. However long it takes, it takes. You're mourning a profound loss, the loss of yourself. There's no closer relationship we have than with ourself. When parents mourn for years and children miss their parents for decades, why wouldn't you grieve and miss yourself for years? And when health care professionals, friends, and family have continually told you to look at the positive and prevented you from grieving and when you're doing it on your own because it's not safe with your community, you'll probably find it tough to start. Excuses to not start or to take a break will crop up. That's OK. You're not procrastinating; you're grieving in therapeutic doses.

But be mindful that breaks don't turn into a permanent stall. Momentum keeps us going and avoids the feat of having to overcome the Go button deficit to start up again after a too-long hiatus. **As for not starting this process, set an appointment with yourself with an audio alarm you can't ignore.**

Reward yourself every time you work through your grief, no matter if it's five minutes or five hours. You weren't able to grieve when your pre-injury self died. But you are now. That's huge!

When you've finished your eulogy, present it out loud like at a funeral. Your presentation may be to a therapist or to a mirror. When done, file it away in an album or post it on your blog. Don't destroy it. Other people's negative opinions on it don't matter. Your eulogy is an homage to yourself. It's sacred work you've done. Treat it as such.

Say A Blessing

You've talked about your old self. Revisited memories and photos. Written stories and a eulogy. Placed your eulogy in a place that reflects its sacredness. You've said au revoir—goodbye until we meet again—to your pre-injury self.

Now it's time to face your new self. Right now, you may feel angst about your new self and your new self changing again and again as you treat your neurons until effective treatments have healed your brain as much as possible. Parts of your pre-injury self may return to merge into your new self. That's why this Action Plan is au revoir, not bye forever.

Action Plan: Saying Au Revoir to You

But before you face your new self, say a blessing on your pre-injury self. Thank them for the life they gave you. Admire their achievements in your blessing. Compliment them on their relationships. And tell them they'll always be in your heart as you move into the final and concurrent Step Five—treating your neurons.

Neurons **HEALING**
Brain restoring
Creates a **NEW**
SELF

Step Five

TREATING YOUR NEURONS

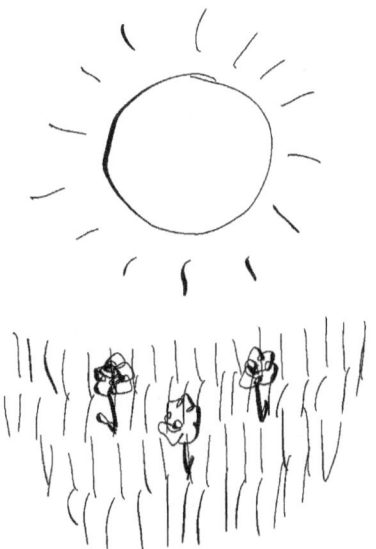

CHAPTER 24

BRAIN-BASED UNDERSTANDING

We're in a transition phase of medical understanding of the brain and brain injury. The traditional way sees brain injury through a subjective DSM lens of symptoms, even when MRI and/or CT show physical damage. The modern way is brain based.

The brain-based perspective sees symptoms as outward manifestations of brain injury, not DSM categories; once neurostimulation or neuromodulation therapies heal the damage, the symptoms vanish—just like once you heal a broken bone, the limb functions pretty much as before the break.

Thomas Insel, the former director of the USA's National Institute of Mental Health, wrote in 2013:

> "While DSM has been described as a 'Bible' for the field, it is, at best, a dictionary, creating a set of labels and defining each. The strength of each of the editions of DSM has been 'reliability'—each edition has ensured that clinicians use the same terms in the same ways. The weakness is its lack of validity. Unlike our definitions of ischemic heart disease, lymphoma, or AIDS, the DSM diagnoses are based on a consensus about clusters of

clinical symptoms, not any objective laboratory measure. In the rest of medicine, this would be equivalent to creating diagnostic systems based on the nature of chest pain or the quality of fever. Indeed, symptom-based diagnosis, once common in other areas of medicine, has been largely replaced in the past half century as we have understood that symptoms alone rarely indicate the best choice of treatment. Patients with mental disorders deserve better."

From John Horgan, Psychiatry in Crisis! Mental Health Director Rejects Psychiatric "Bible" and Replaces With Nothing, Scientific American, 4 May 2013 https://blogs.scientificamerican.com/cross-check/psychiatry-in-crisis-mental-health-director-rejects-psychiatric-bible-and-replaces-with-nothing/

The brain-based lens assesses brain activity using well-researched, objective tests such as qEEG, evoke potentials, SPECT, and diffuse tensor imaging (DTI).

These tests show which areas of the brain are working, which have slowed, which are disconnected or too connected, and so on. They show the brain's overall power, which is a measure of neuro-fatigue. They explain symptoms neurophysiologically.

Although more and more clinics are switching to brain-based assessments, standard medical care continues to rely on subjective symptom and DSM-based questionnaires. Unfortunately, they allow patients to believe the only objective tests are MRIs or CT scans; if these tests show nothing, then they either dismiss patients, offer strategies and rest, or provide ineffective "cognitive therapy." They don't offer tests that show brain activity.

"What make brain injuries particularly challenging — outside of the fact it is the epicentre for human functioning — is they are difficult to diagnose, relying heavily on self-reported symptoms."

From Shannon Devine, Toronto Star, 13 June 2022 https://www.thestar.com/opinion/contributors/2022/06/13/there-are-15-million-canadians-living-with-a-brain-injury-we-can-do-more-to-help-them-recover.html

Those clinics using the brain-based lens to diagnose and treat brain injury don't rely on self-reported symptoms for diagnosis; they conduct qEEG or evoke potentials or SPECT to determine what needs treating.

Once we're exposed to brain-based understanding of the brain and brain injury, mistrust creeps in to our relationship with a traditional psychiatrist or neurologist who refers to brain injury symptoms as mood disorders and DSM categories instead of neurophysiological changes such as too little beta brainwave activity or too much busy brain. DSM-biased specialists may refuse to learn about and switch to the brain-based lens. For them, the DSM has been around for decades as a reliable medical assessment of psychiatric conditions.

The DSM is familiar but unilluminating.

unfamiliar brain-based assessments illuminate brain injury

For example, we understand depression as a DSM category requiring medications. But the brain-based lens sees depression as a change in brain activity in particular regions that neurostimulation therapies can rebalance. The brain-based lens understands that brain injury can injure these areas, thus creating the same lopsided brain activity as depression. Specialists can permanently heal it through either the same or different neurostimulation therapies. Here, the diagnosis of depression is inappropriate because *the cause is injury*, even though the symptoms seem identical.

Symptoms cannot pinpoint the location of damage; cannot explain the feelings of chaos in the brain; provide no understanding of brain fog, non-responsiveness, and so on; and cannot be the basis for an effective treatment plan that leads to dramatic healing of the injury.

You may end up feeling abandoned to your brain injury, knowing that if they'd used the brain-based lens, you'd have had a chance at full recovery or at least life-changing healing. Yet, you may also continue to see them because so few medicare-covered psychiatrists treat brain injury and because they still listen to you with compassion.

LEARN MORE

"Medicine is both an art and a science. In objective testing, humans cannot bias the results through subconscious cues, which even well-trained specialists can give. Brains supporting brains does not occur during objective tests as the specialist is not near the client during the testing. And objective tests do not depend on subjective answers to symptom-type questions." See Introduction to Diagnosis of Brain Injury for more information at https://concussionisbraininjury.com/diagnosis/introduction-to-diagnosis-of-brain-injury/.

CHAPTER 25

LESSONS I'VE LEARNED

Empowering Yourself

This book so far has been about facing up to your losses, healing your grief, learning to live with the awfulness of brain-injury affected relationships, seeing your gifts, and most of all recognizing that the creative force—God or the cosmos—wants you here. Is glad you're here. Wants you healed.

I'm hoping you feel more ready to find and receive effective treatments to treat your neurons.

As the daughter of an eminent clinician-researcher and being a prodigious reader before my brain injury, I naturally gravitated to discussing with all my health care providers my health issues and probable courses of action. I was used to my long-time GP (now deceased) asking my opinion, listening to my knowledge before deciding the next step in my health care. His ability to remember what I told him always astounded me. My father had a similar memory for his patients and for current research findings. My father treated patients with incurable complex gastrointestinal diseases and developed home total parenteral nutrition to improve their health and quality of life (see *Lifeliner* in Readings section). Both my father and GP attended medical college when physiology and anatomy were the foundations of medical knowledge and house calls the norm. Medicine fascinated both. They read widely to satiate their curiosity, to change their "I don't know" answers to here's what may help. Perhaps that's why they had well-developed memory muscles, an even-more-important skill today with our increasing knowledge, breadth of complex treatments, and increasingly empowered patients. Perhaps that's also why they treated their patients as human beings like family, not insurance codes.

Mine and others' traumatic brain injuries strained my GP's resources. Yet I could still count on him to keep abreast of my brain injury treatments, to know what blood tests to order and how to read X-rays; to not dismiss me if I disagreed with him; to discuss with me why he believed his particular recommendation was the right one while respecting and incorporating my gained knowledge and self-insights; and to consider carefully which specialists to refer me to. He was a family physician who accepted and respected patient empowerment before that phrase was invented while, at the same time, took responsibility for guiding and directing my patient care.

I miss that security.

Kamal Jethwani, MD, MPH and Jodi Sperber, PhD wrote in December 2017 "Who Gives Us the Right to 'Empower' Patients?":

> "Giving power to users means that health care providers reduce our own power in the relationship. Are we ready for that? If so, health care organizations and individual providers should consider using words and language more appropriate for our role in the users' care, such as coach, guide, counselor, or advocate. These words uphold the specialized nature of our expertise, but also equalize the relationship somewhat. We could also consider adopting a more passive persona, to correct the pendulum that is currently swung too much on the other end."

It is one thing to have an equal say about my health care; it's another to have to learn medicine and drive it. With a brain injury, no less! The latter is the current situation you and I find ourselves in. Having to both coordinate our care and learn enough to drive our treatments overwhelms and paralyzes.

Patient empowerment should be about working in concert with one's physicians, not about making every single medical decision and coordinating care. Excellent health care ought to be about the physician bringing to the table their expertise and the patient bringing to the table their self-knowledge and the two working together. Yet here we are doing both.

> "Jethwani and Sperber defined clinical needs as accurate diagnoses and treatment options. Right now, standard medical care provides neither for brain injury, and that's a problem. They argued that health care providers should not only satisfy these clinical needs but also extend beyond them to educate and to address social determinants of health, social support, abilities, preferences, fears, cultures, and attitudes."
>
> *From* Who Is Responsible for a Patient's Health Care?, Psychology Today, 16 Sep 2019 https://www.psychology-today.com/ca/blog/concussion-is-brain-injury/201909/who-is-responsible-patients-health-care/

Until GPs, psychiatrists, neurologists, and rehab move to brain-based understanding and treatment of brain injury, we will have to support and rely on each other to share knowledge to find the treatments we need to heal our brains.

That's why I created https://concussionisbraininjury.com and wrote this book: to give you the tools to find accurate diagnoses and learn how to assess which neurostimulation treatments work. Hopefully, these resources will empower you.

Taking a Step Back:
My Psychology Perspective

Once upon a time, I knew a philandering man. With his cheeky grin and charm, his arms were never empty. A bevy of young women followed him wherever he went. Easy promises and big ideas slid off his tongue; as I laughed with him, I believed not a word. As he grew up, his character emerged through his surface charm; some of us noticed how he quietly gave dignity to the elderly who couldn't toilet themselves. Yet his empty promises and profligate ways lead to labels of unfit, unreliable, a guileful personality. The labels gave some a reason to shun him, although he helped vulnerable people out in ways his "betters" wouldn't.

People chose two ways to react to him. Anger, frustration, and resentment or acceptance. The former abandoned him in his time of need. Those who accepted him for who he was, someone with charm and empty promises who also served the helpless, didn't allow labels and anger to cast a wedge between him and them. How do you and the people around you react to troublesome people? Labelling and anger? Or having a clear-eyed view of them and keeping mithra alive between you?

At the University of Toronto, I studied psychology to find out what makes people tick. I wanted to understand the inexplicable. I applied for and was accepted into the specialist program, which is more onerous than a major. You're required to take every course in abnormal psychology (as it was called then). The thought excited me! From all my courses, only once did a course section leave me puzzled and disappointed.

That was the section on organic brain issues, including brain injury.

I read the required textbook cover to cover. At the end of one fascinating chapter, I read a page on organic brain injury. I turned the page. The next chapter stared back at me. I flipped the page back in disbelief. That was it? That was everything known on such a substantial topic? One page? Yup. Decades later, God answered my disappointment by giving me personal experience, research, and learnings through my own brain injury. I never would have asked for nor have imagined such a way to satisfy my curiosity on this subject!

We with brain injury are seen as troublesome, lazy, toxic people, for the neuroscience-related fields of medicine and psychology have expanded little since I studied at the University of Toronto. Although they've adopted neuroplasticity within their understanding, they relegate it to meditation and such-like. Only individual clinics, researchers, and specialists have broadened their practices into brain-based understanding of neuroplasticity and brain injury.

I've talked about how God loves you, how you're a wanted part of Nature, and now I want to approach healing ourself and our neurons from a different perspective.

Action Plan: What Matters to You?

Find time to sit in your quiet place, prepare with deep breathing, decide on your reward, and have ready your stress busters. Reward yourself for spending even five minutes on this Action Plan. Five minutes is better than zero. Not completing it is better than not starting. Reward yourself for starting!

Open the new notebook *Hello Healing*. On the first page, write the title, "What Matters to Me?"

List without thinking everything that matters to you. You can be as general or as specific as you want. Include your inmost desires, the ones you try not to think about because you don't know how you'll achieve them.

Then write the heading "Social." Under it, list the people you want in your life, the ones who nurture you or you depend on. By this time, you hopefully will no longer desire to spend time with people who drain you of energy and demand you be like your old self. If you find you're still wishing instead of living in the reality of these relationships, return to Step Two, Wishes Are Not Reality Action Plan.

Reflect on the People in Your Life

Think about how each of the people left in your life affects your energy.
- Do they drain your energy or give you energy?
- Do they keep you in your injured state, have a neutral effect, or encourage you to seek healing and better treatments?

Spend as little time as possible with stuck people who label you. If you depend on them, tune out their criticisms and judgements. Be like the fictional character Nero Wolfe: don't let others shift you from what works to heal, improve your energy, and keep you as healthy as possible. More on Nero Wolfe later in this chapter.

Remember: any time someone fibs about qEEG, that it's a waste of money, or insists brain biofeedback appointments don't work, say "OK" and leave the room. Or if you're so fatigued, you can't move, say nothing, close your eyes, remember neurostimulation works to restore neurons and reset microglia, patience reaps rewards, and you're working to heal yourself. That which created you wants you to thrive. It's about what matters to you not to them. And you want your brain back.

Action Plan: Set Yourself Up For Success

The problem with traditional rehab is that it presents cognitive strategies as actually being able to do cognitive work. Using highlighters, notes in margins, pacing as reading strategies doesn't lead to you being able to read. Eventually, we cannot avoid the truth of that. When it becomes apparent, it feels like we failed at both rehab and reading.

Set Your Health As Your Top Priority to Succeed

From the start, I set myself up for success. I had enough experience with illness and injury to know that I had to recover first before I tried to resume work. I had to set my health as my top priority. Without health, everything else eventually falters. Work soon lets you go, friends become distant, and family blames you. That leads to feeling like a failure.

Success comes from following two concurrent roads: staying within your limits of brain injury while pursuing neurostimulation therapies to restore brain function, including cognitions.

Instead of trying to be normal, trying to live as if you don't have a brain injury, focus on what matters most to you. From your What Matters To You? list, choose one function, skill, hobby, or volunteering goal and consider the obstacles to doing it, what success in it looks like, and how you'd achieve that success.

On a fresh page, list the obstacles in your *Hello Healing* notebook.

Title a new page with each obstacle and list how you'll overcome it. But unlike rehab, reflect as well on what brain function you need to restore so that you can achieve success.

For example, maybe you want to write. But you can't concentrate for long, can't stick to commitments, and you have energy only for an hour a week. You have two concurrent roads to writing. The first road uses strategies, the kind of thing rehab would teach you; the second involves receiving brain biofeedback, an effective neurostimulation treatment.

Road One. A blog lets you write without requiring you to commit to writing to someone else's deadlines. Set up a blog schedule of less than once a week. Set your timer for a half hour. Write whatever you can in that half hour. When the timer goes off, stop. Stretch. Eat that half cookie made with whole grain flour. Return. Set your timer for 15 minutes and revise your post or add an image. When your timer goes off, publish it. Tick it off in your calendar as done. Put a gold star emoticon next to it. Reward yourself with your favourite TV show.

set your schedule and timer for less than what you can do →

Setting your timer for less than your maximum capacity is how you set yourself up for success. You don't want to push yourself. When you sit down to write, you'll probably end up continuing after your timer alarms. But since you set your timer for less than what you can do on average, going over time will less likely cause you to crash and more likely to blog regularly. Keep in mind that seasonal changes and unexpected events may kibosh your plans for a few weeks. That's OK. That's the nature of brain injury. And because it's your blog, you're not failing anyone, including yourself.

Road Two. While staying on Road One, also find and attend a clinic that conducts qEEG and evoke potentials tests (see the chapter Neurostimulation Therapies Work in this Step). These tests will show the specialist where to apply brain biofeedback to restore concentration, improve stamina, and increase energy. As your neurons regrow and rewire, you'll gradually transform Road One. At the end of the treatment protocols, you'll be able to blog longer, more often, and regularly without needing timers and rest times before and after.

Being Overwhelmed by Treatments and Healing

Brain injury overwhelms in two ways. The injury itself requires juggling a lot of medical, health, personal daily life, and social life events. And since our brain doesn't work well, events or situations or people can overwhelm our injured neurons. Knowing we can become easily overwhelmed is the first step to dealing with it.

After a few years of being alone, you'll have learnt what overwhelms you, but neurostimulation therapies that speed up healing and restore as much brain function as possible bring new challenges. Challenges encompass returning emotions, cognitions, strength, stamina, energy, and so on; relearning the norm for each of these areas or adapting to significant improvement takes time and guidance. Without guidance, we will figure it out through trial and error, but it'll take longer and include hard bumps on the road. Although it seemed to me like the road contained endless bumps, they did smooth out. The most important first step upon realizing our brain is overwhelmed is to step away and step into what places the least burden on your brain. That may include watching an animated movie on Netflix or sitting on a park bench to watch the passing parade. In addition, use a short alpha protocol or a standard SMR one on the audiovisual entrainment device. Resting the brain, distracting your mind, not napping, is how to recharge.

take time out when you're overwhelmed →

You want to avoid napping outside of a regular afternoon rest time. The newest suggestion for optimum rest time is to rest seven hours after you get up, and nap only for about a half hour and no more.

rest longer but don't sleep longer than 30 minutes during the day →

You want to stay in the world but not let it burden you. That way you know you're still part of mithra but you're also protecting yourself and your brain's resources. From such a restful but engaging place, you build up your sense of competence and continue your brain's path to healing.

Self-Advocacy Sucks

I grew up in a medical household; socialized with my father's residents, Fellows, and colleagues; lived with my mother and sister for three months with my father's research partner's family while our family home was being renovated; and stayed with his first mentor Dr. N Coghill's family when visiting England. In short, I viewed physicians as my social equals, knowing more than patients, and I knew how to spot an excellent one versus those who coasted. I met many of my father's patients and wrote on one, Judy Taylor, who was the first person in the world to live without eating. Taylor and my father's medical pioneering story is up there with Banting and Best, more known outside of Canada than here in Toronto where the groundbreaking work happened. Through my research for *Lifeliner: The Judy Taylor Story*, I learnt how Taylor thrived. The four essentials included:

1. A person has a goal and strong will to live.
2. A medical team provides care and support that a patient can count on to heal them.
3. Social support.
4. Faith.

I applied these lessons to my own life after I suffered a brain injury. Unfortunately, I had little social support and no advocacy from my family or friends. After several years, I realized that medical care of brain injury was the opposite of the care my father Dr. Khursheed N. Jeejeebhoy and his team gave their total parenteral nutrition patients like Taylor. If I was going to get better, I had to search alone for treatments that worked and be forthright with the health care professionals when their treatments weren't working.

In fits and starts, I learnt to overcome my prejudice that health care professionals know more than patients about their condition. I struggled to navigate around my injured brain's inability to express my thoughts well enough to communicate my needs. Desperation to recover my cognitions drove the latter.

self-advocacy is easier without affect →

Self-advocating was what I did to get my brain back. Having no affect helped me. The solitariness of pushing back against professional ignorance and pushing for better treatments didn't create excruciatingly high levels of emotional pain. The odd time my affect turned on before turning off again kept the pain brief. And so I could focus on finding what I needed, sticking to the fatiguing brain biofeedback treatments without home support, going from physician to physician in a search of answers for my high body temperature that had landed me in the ER, developing my hypothalamus fix when I received no help for it, and taking advantage of every opportunity to relearn to write and to write books.

When brain biofeedback gamma brainwave enhancement therapy began to heal my affect, I found it more and more difficult to advocate for myself. A decade of self-advocacy had also psychologically and physically exhausted me. Self-advocacy requires pushing through many damaged cognitions. From having to remember how neurostimulation worked so I could counter the no-research crowd to navigating others' fears around an unknown therapy to having the emotional courage to say bluntly your therapy isn't working and this is what I need. The emotional toll was horrendous.

Thinking about the toll, I wonder why anyone advises people with brain injury—those whose cognitions are damaged—to self-advocate instead of advocating for them.

To Self-Advocate or Not Self-Advocate?

Unfortunately, you and I being alone with our brain injury, have only two choices: self-advocate or moulder in our injury with no hope ever again. But I feel your suffering as you embark on self-advocacy and, through my writings, am here to reassure you you're not alone. I and many others have gone before you to smooth down the bumpy road.

Education creates advocates in the community and empowers people with brain injury to self-advocate as much as they can, when they can.

LEARN MORE

> I hope this Step will help you find a way to self-advocate with your eyes wide open to its reality. Perhaps you'll find someone to advocate alongside you by sharing with them this book, my *Psychology Today* blog https://www.psychologytoday.com/ca/blog/concussion-is-brain-injury, my website https://concussionisbraininjury.com, and memoir *Concussion Is Brain Injury: Treating the Neurons and Me*.

Be Like Nero Wolfe

Nero Wolfe, Rex Stout's fictional detective, is famous for his rules. Nothing interferes with Wolfe's routine. He brooks no discussion of business during meal times. Food is to be enjoyed. Meal time is for rivetting conversation. The hours of 9:00 to 11:00 AM and 4:00 to 6:00 PM are for his hobby, tending his 10,000 orchids. He never leaves his house, except under duress.

Be like Nero Wolfe! Set up a routine that optimizes your brain function and fills your day with a mix of pleasure and necessary appointments. A routine will conserve your energy to use it for the things that matter to you. Doing what matters most to you, not what others say should matter to you, enhances energy. Unless and until you're able to access appropriate diagnostics and effective neurostimulation therapies to treat your neurons, some strategies are necessary.

the most important strategy is energy conservation ➔

You learnt about pacing during rehab. But pacing isn't really about energy conservation. It's about being able to do something, anything, for a little while. It's part of energy conservation. Energy conservation is about being able to function in the way you want to, as best as you can, daily.

Energy Conservation

What's more important to you?
1. Maintaining social relationships no matter the cost to you and your brain?
2. Or treating your neurons and healing your person so that you can gain the life you want?

Energy conservation is about making this decision and using your energy towards what matters most to you.

The second choice, treating your neurons, may in time allow you to focus on the first choice, on social relationships after you've regained conversational and social abilities. Think of treating your neurons as being in a virtual hospital. In-patients aren't thinking about their social life; they're using all their resources to get better and leave the hospital. After discharge, they resume work, play, and their social life. We're the same.

Nero Wolfe Excels at Focusing on What Matters to Him

For Nero Wolfe, his detective business brings in the money and exercises his brain so that he can savour good food and keep orchids. His routine allows him to pursue what matters most to him with the minimum of anxiety. Wolfe is an agoraphobic—he fears roads, cars, chairs too small for his bulk. He creates a social life in the men who lives with him in his home:

Archie, the narrator of the novels and Wolfe's man of action. Fritz, his cook, who he creates elaborate meals with. And Theodore, the man who tends his orchids and rarely interacts with Fritz or Archie.

Wolfe conserves his energy for what matters most to him, surrounded by people who care about him, support him, and love his eccentricities, though at times they aggravate them.

Wolfe knows to toss out people who impose judgements on him and force him to expend precious energy to withstand them. He doesn't care what others think of him. But then, he's not isolated. Perhaps knowing you're cherished by that which created you will surge in new strength and free you to conserve your energy. Return to Step One if you need reinforcing and reassuring that you're lovable and loved. That your desires matter. That the one who created you is glad you're here and wants you to pursue what matters to you.

Stagnation versus Energy Giving

What are you using your energy on and for? People who keep you stagnant or those who help you heal? Treating your neurons and retraining skills and talents you want back, or doing what others want you to do?

Those who deride you, criticize your brain injury effects, or expect you to socialize in the way you used to before your injury, stagnates you. But there is no return to pre-injury status quo. We are not the same. The only way to heal brain injury is through radical adoption of innovative treatments. To do that, we have to alter our perspective on what's good medicine.

Is Your Medical Care Stagnating You?

What's it like to alter your perspective against authority and parental figures? A story. I grew up in a medical household, headed by a physician who achieved three professorships at the University of Toronto, developed home artificial feeding—total parenteral nutrition—that saves lives every year, and became world famous for his nutritional discoveries and clinical care. I didn't have a family doctor until my twenties. Although my father innovated medicine all the time, he and my mother, a nurse, raised me with a certain idea of medicine, that science superseded ancient ways. And so when I suffered a seatbelt injury in my 1991 car crash that rendered my dominant arm almost non-functional, I looked to modern medical science for answers. I received prednisone injections in my neck. They rid me of the daily migraines but didn't restore my arm function. What to do? The treating physician referred me to a physiatrist at a teaching hospital in 1993. That referral challenged my assumptions of good medicine.

logic and reason take the limits off established medical thought

People consider me stubborn with strong opinions. But I also have a logical mind, and my parents and university taught me to think critically. I reach my opinions only after careful thought, with a willingness to change my mind when new facts appear. I liked the fact the physiatrist used objective tests to measure my arm's nerve function, even though the tests hurt like hell. Unlike a neurologist I'd seen earlier, he didn't dismiss me based on normal muscle function test results; he listened and used his brain to search for other possibilities. I think that neurologist's attitude reflects what I find so reprehensible in the medical profession: those who should know better and do better in diagnosing our nervous systems and brains, self-restrict their thinking, are unwilling to listen to the patient, and resist leaving their familiar approach in order to diagnose and treat significant problems that impede work and reduce quality of life.

This physiatrist was one of the few who did.

The physiatrist found my ulnar nerve wasn't conducting and reviewed the test results with me. He presented me with two options: nerve surgery or acupuncture.

I knew that nerve surgery was more likely to compound the problem than help. I'd heard enough about this kind of surgery from my father to stay away from it. *But acupuncture?!* Back then, medicine and the public viewed acupuncture as an ancient art with no evidence behind it. I thought acupuncture didn't work—it's not based on science. It only worked because people "believe" in it; the placebo effect meant they saw healing where none existed because they believed it to be so. But I have a logical mind and I use my reason.

I'd eliminated surgery as an option. So, like Sherlock Holmes, once you dismiss the impossible, whatever is left, no matter how improbable, you try. I chose acupuncture, despite my fear of needles and my habit of going white at blood labs. The physiatrist mused about whom to send me to for acupuncture, whether it was better to wait for the true expert or have me seen immediately. He chose the waiting option. Thank goodness!

open minds break barriers

I had an open mind insofar as I was willing to give it a try. Plus, I was desperate. I stepped way outside my box of what made up good medical care, and, unlike when my mother accompanied me to the blood lab, no one came with me to hold me up through my fear of needles. I doubted it'd work.

Alone in Trying New Medicine

When the acupuncturist put the needles in my skin, I felt like my body was a map of magnetic compass needles that suddenly went from chaos to all pointing in the same direction. Astounding. Definitely not an effect based on any belief I had! I changed my mind about acupuncture. I began to question the infallibility of modern science as having the only answers. Just because we don't currently understand how something works doesn't mean that ancient peoples were wrong.

Specialists Who Break Out of Their Boxes

The moral of this story is you want to find specialists willing to think beyond their established medicine box in order to help you. Specialists who learn only because they have to and stick to familiar territory keep you stuck in brain injury and drain you. Find specialists who will actually treat your neurons, for they will give you energy.

Spend Energy on Healing Appointments

Our medical appointments drain us of energy for the rest of the day. Minimizing them helps conserve energy. Discern which appointments matter and which ones can be folded into others so that you see fewer health care professionals on fewer days. This will free up energy for what matters to you.

For example, is it worth seeing psychiatrists who see you only for 15-minute medication checks but consume an entire day's worth of energy? If your family physician can prescribe these medications, then see them for medication checks at your regular appointments, for at least it's one less person to see. (With brain injury, I assume you see your family physician regularly, although I'm aware there's a crisis in family medicine. For some, psychiatrists provide regular care, in which case, using your energy to see them is more appropriate.) Alternatively, maybe see the medication-check psychiatrist virtually. That way, you don't have to give up an entire day's worth of energy to see a psychiatrist who can't be bothered to do more than monitor your prescription and/or check your bloodwork results.

Meanwhile, use your energy to attend appointments with neurostimulation specialists and, as those therapies radically heal you, decrease or eventually eliminate the standard medical care ones that don't do much for you.

Energy conservation means using as little as possible on what's unavoidable and shifting it to what treats your neurons and gives you meaning.

CHAPTER 26

EMOTIONAL COURAGE

Facing the Boulders to Treating Your Brain

"One night I dreamt of boulders rising out of the water. Behind and to the left and right of me lay the land. Amorphous green trees surrounded me. The black, glistening boulders loomed out of the calm water of deceptive depths to block my escape. Every time I clambered over one, another would rise up ahead of me. Always before me were ragged rows of water-rubbed round boulders and rocks, their blackness both glistened and sucked in all the light.

I couldn't escape.

The depth of the water beyond the boulders terrified me, for I didn't know what lay beneath or if a boulder would suddenly pop up. I awoke."

From Concussion Is Brain Injury: Treating the Neurons and Me.

The biggest boulder to anyone trying to heal their brain injury is physicians not learning and adopting neurostimulation and neuromodulation treatments.

> "My dog trotted behind me as I headed to the bathroom, hoping I'd given myself enough time to get to my psychologist's for what he called neurofeedback, but time meant nothing to me. I really didn't care if I was early or late until I was there. It was so far into the future, the only thing that mattered was the now....The elephant was on my chest, but the neurofeedback my psychologist provided awaited me. Oh my God, I hope I get to have it! I didn't have it every week. Some weeks, my psychologist decided I needed to do visualization exercises instead, and I was unable to open my mouth to ask him for the neurofeedback when it looked like I wouldn't get it. But I really, really wanted that neurofeedback, that light and sound show, as I called it. It gave me energy. It helped me think. Please, God, let him give me the feedback."
>
> *From* Concussion Is Brain Injury: Treating the Neurons and Me.

Fortunately, the first psychologist I saw after my car crash used an effective treatment, one he called neurofeedback and is now called audiovisual entrainment. The problem was that I received it, at best, once weekly when I should have had a home unit for daily use.

So when a new psychologist advised me to buy Mind Alive's home unit, I snapped it up.

Maybe one day, every psychologist and psychiatrist will have learnt about neurostimulation, will introduce it to their clients and patients, and provide us with info on where to purchase home medical devices. Until then, we must find the internal strength and emotional courage to purchase it ourself despite the naysayers and lack of physician adoption. I'm hoping at this point in the book, you feel empowered to pursue treating your neurons, realizing that if you don't, no one else will...unless you're lucky enough to have a medicare-covered psychologist or psychiatrist who prescribes and/or treats brain injury this way.

The Power of Speaking to Creation

One way towards strengthening ourself to break barriers is prayer. It's become fashionable to mock prayers as useless religious claptrap. I grew up confused by prayer rules. Pray in the morning before work, but don't ask what the adult is praying. Pray prayers at church from a book without thinking. Kneel beside the bed and pray from a pretty, little children's prayer book. Pray the Lord's Prayer. Except for the last, all these ritualistic prayers pinged off me. Either I had no idea what I was supposed to say or I found my mind wandered. Perhaps because of Jesus saying hello to me when I was six, over the decades, my prayers became conversations with Jesus, God, or the Holy Spirit. After my brain injury, the Lord's Prayer transformed itself in my mind. It sparked a conversation about what was bothering me the most. I became used to not finishing it, so intent was I on talking with God about the latest setback and people important to me. Prayer activates mithra.

After my brain injury, I'd walk home alone after rehab, exhausted, worried my legs would stop from no muscle power before I reached my front door. I'd look up at the beautiful Canadian blue sky for my sole gratitude moment, and I'd find Jesus walking beside me, listening intently. It's not like I can see him with my eyeballs. It's more like a sense when you know someone is thinking about you and you see them appear in your mind's eye. Or when you feel someone observing you. Just like we talk out our worries with a best friend, so, too, we can talk to God or Jesus about what's bothering us. In talking anytime, anywhere, we feel less alone and become stronger in pursuing a radical path.

In 2011, B. Waldron-Perrine and colleagues studied faith and rehab outcomes among African-American men with traumatic brain injury and their knowledgeable significant others. Although religious activity had no predictive value, a person's personal connection with a higher power improved life satisfaction, reduced distress, and predicted a better functional outcome.

prayer enhances interpersonal connection, mithra ➤

Zarathustra taught we walk hand in hand with God. That doesn't mean I do all the work or God does all the work. We work collaboratively, within our own spheres of influence and ability. With brain injury, I needed extra help, like the image of Jesus carrying us when we're helpless.

God sent me help when it was available and when I dropped off the end of my rope and quit. I don't know why I had to reach desperate depths before God answered. But while humans repeated their mantra of get on with your life, God eventually connected me with effective, healing help. Jesus walked with me, attentive, non-judgemental, kind. The Holy Spirit kicked me out of bed when neuro-fatigue fastened me under the sheets and despair gripped my heart. Jesus's spirit guided me away from danger, overcame my fear of costly, non-standard treatments, and told me where to next. I prayed for first-draft writing every time I sat down to write *Lifeliner*, for I didn't have the energy, stamina, cognition, or patience to write multiple drafts like before my brain injury. God assented. Having regular conversations, regular complaint sessions, regular thankful thoughts for blue skies and past help, allowed me to connect and receive. God never scolded me for complaining too much or my anger or quitting multiple times. That merciful, kind relationship gave me emotional courage to get back up and going again.

I don't know if conversations with Nature, with the vastness of the universe, would have the same effect, but enhancing mithra—our interconnections—can help. Talking to a tree, communing with the stars, asking a squirrel what they're chittering about, telling cats to knock off fighting, could enhance the connection with our world, making us feel less alone and so less distressed.

Relationships require regular conversations. I believe conversing regularly with God, Jesus, or the universe enhances mithra and helps with emotional courage.

LEARN MORE

> "Recovering from brain injury is more than relearning to walk and read, it's also about finding your new identity, discovering a new or renewed purpose, trying to create meaning out of catastrophic suffering so that one can thrive again. Faith undergirds the latter." For more on this subject, see https://www.psychologytoday.com/ca/blog/concussion-is-brain-injury/202104/does-faith-serve-purpose-after-brain-injury.

Action Plan: Developing Emotional Courage

"Emotional courage is the willingness to feel. And it's the driving force behind anything important that we accomplish." Peter Bregman, quoted in *Forbes*, Why Emotional Courage Is So Essential To Leadership, Kathy Caprino, 6 July 2018. I'd add that after brain injury, it's the courage to go beyond the standard medical practice of strategies and rest to obtain healing for your brain.

It's true that emotions enhance thinking, as I discovered when my affect returned. But you can still have emotional courage in the absence of affect. Bregman continues:

> "There's something you don't want to feel. Maybe it's the possibility of conflict. Or the other person's defensiveness. Or their anger. Or your own anger or defensiveness. I'm not sure what it is that you might have to feel—but the risk of feeling it stops you. It stops all of us. That's why emotional courage is so important to following through on what we care most about."

For us with brain injury, it's not so much the feeling of conflict as the inability to handle it. Without necessary cognitions, conflict with another ends up defeating us. Anger may also paralyze us into silence as I wrote in the revised edition of *Concussion Is Brain Injury: Treating the Neurons and Me*:

> "A second hidden anger issue is response to others' anger.
>
> A neurotypical person would at least step back from in-your-face, sudden, top-volume yelling. After my brain injury, I don't. Although I startle when a squirrel bounces by, I don't even flinch when a stranger yells in my face. My brain blanks. My body freezes. In response, people either leave or begin to speak to me slowly and carefully like I'm extremely stupid. But none have ana-

lyzed why this happens or treated the involved damaged areas so that I can be safe."

How do you find the emotional courage to pursue brain injury healing when it'll lead to conflict with standard medical practice and with loved ones who believe strategies and rest are treatments and neurostimulation is a scam with no research to back it? (There are thousands of research studies, starting over a century ago. Ignoring the research or not looking for it doesn't mean there's none.)

Finding Emotional Courage

I hope this book is helping you regrow your self-worth, to know that the force that created you is always on the side of healing your broken neurons. But you may not yet feel self-confident. Bregman suggests one way to build confidence:

> "identify where you are comfortable being different than the people around you....It may be something that seems insignificant to you—like eating differently than the people you're with (maybe you're kosher or vegetarian, or hate blue cheese—and you're comfortable holding that line even when other people are making different choices). Think about those situations and feel what it feels like to stand in your certainty, in your willingness to be with people and be different from them. Feel that sense of self.
>
> As you notice that place in your body, you can then begin to apply it to other areas of your life."

Self-confidence and self-worth strengthen us to face conflict when we pursue treatments for our neurons.

Using Aids to Compensate

Since brain injury impairs cognitions like decision-making and memory, you may need compensating aids to help you manage conflict until you've attended and completed effective treatments. Besides using silence as I wrote in Resistance Is Not Futile in Step Two or reading preset responses as a way to handle criticism and judgement, you can also use two decision-making tools I've found useful.

Decision-Making Strategies

Begin by talking the problem over with people you trust or your local Help line. If you feel driven to talk it over with everyone, don't worry about it. It's how you are. Recurring decisions can be decided once then done the same way every time. For example, always buy four apples of the same kind.

In your *Hello Healing* notebook, on a fresh page, write what you need to decide on. Then use one of the two methods below. If you're still unsure, set an alarm for a month later to look at it then and redo either the Decision Tree or SOLVE method. If you still cannot decide, reset the alarm for two weeks hence and repeat.

Decision Tree

Draw a vertical line down the middle of the page and at the top of the page, title each column with decision options. For example, I created a decision tree **to decide** whether or not to travel to England. I titled the columns "Visit England" and "Don't Visit England." Draw two vertical lines down the page, one underneath each option. Write "Pros" and "Cons" at the top of the columns for each option. Now list supportive points in each column without thinking. For example, the pros and cons of visiting England, and the pros and cons of not visiting England. When done, you'll notice what stands out. Discuss with your therapist or trusted person if you're still unsure. For me, the biggest con was financial. I asked myself if financial cost overrode the biggest benefit. It didn't, and I found a way to afford it. As a result, I experienced benefits that paid off dramatically in non-financial ways, and the money resolved itself in the end.

SOLVE

SOLVE is an acronym for a method of solving problems or making decisions.

Select the problem.
Observe and define the problem or situation. Question all aspects.
Listen to advice from others about the problem.
Visualize potential solutions and choose one.
Employ the solution and monitor the results.

My therapist told me most people don't like to listen to advice from others. I think we can learn from anyone, and I try to find a trusted person to present my problem to and listen to what they have to say. I may adopt it in whole, in part, or not at all when coming up with solutions.

To use this method, in your *Hello Healing* notebook, write on a fresh page the decision you want to make. Underneath, write the letters of SOLVE vertically, with room between letters to write out your thoughts. Then follow the steps.

- Write out the problem.
- Define it and describe all angles of it.
- Jot down what others advise.
- Note what solutions you see; underline the one you choose.
- Write about how you will employ your chosen solution.
- Note how your chosen solution is working out.

If your solution doesn't work, repeat and choose another solution. You may have to give yourself time to process some of these steps before continuing.

Using Emotional Courage

The third step is to focus on what you want: to treat your injured neurons. Open your *Hello Healing* notebook and write, "I want to regenerate my injured neurons." Perhaps copy it on a post-it note and stick it where you can see it to remind you of this life-changing decision.

Remind yourself that this decision is worth following. It'll be difficult, but the reward will be beyond what your health care providers can imagine for you. Be willing to face the conflict to achieve what matters to you. Taking the risk of facing the conflict will build your emotional courage. But build up to that risk level, especially if the thought of going against the people quails you.

Begin building your emotional courage with something small. Something that feels risky but doesn't contravene standard medical advice. Something where *perceived* risk is *less than* actual risk. Perhaps it's finally to stop drinking alcohol or taking drugs, both of which are bad for brain injury. Or maybe, after being used to eating half a dozen cookies at a time, it's allowing yourself to eat only half a chocolate chip cookie made with whole grain flour after working on your grief or with bibliotherapy, as both a reward and to refuel your brain. Go slowly. Feel the feelings that come up, the way your body reacts, how your brain works, yet don't let those feelings or thoughts stop you. If they do, give yourself time to recover, strengthen yourself, set up rewards for completing before trying again. These feelings will be the same as when you're ready to take the risk of treating your neurons.

When you manage the small risk and feel stronger for it, try a slightly bigger risk, then a bit bigger, and so on until you're able to state firmly that you want your neurons treated and you're willing to do what it takes to have qEEG and evoke potentials and to work at effective neurostimulation treatments.

LEARN MORE

Use the resources in the revised edition of *Concussion Is Brain Injury* and at https://concussionisbraininjury.com to learn about how to treat your neurons, find out what it's like, and restore your brain to the best functionality innovative medical science can achieve today.

Action Plan: Setting Your Treatment Goal

I learnt in my stress management class during neurorehab that a goal improves the outcome.

My Treatment Goal

I wanted to write *Lifeliner: The Judy Taylor Story*, and I wanted to read again.
- Without audiovisual entrainment, I would've stayed stuck in zombie mode.
- Without brain biofeedback, I wouldn't have been able to regain my attention span in order to do anything.
- Without brain biofeedback, I wouldn't have been able to write *Lifeliner*, my first goal.
- Without audiovisual entrainment and cranioelectrical stimulation, I wouldn't have been able to significantly improve my body temperature regulation and sleep.
- Without transcranial direct current stimulation (battery-powered tDCS), I wouldn't have regained normal conversational skills.
- Without LORETA brain biofeedback, I wouldn't have had my brain work more efficiently and quickly, allowing me to socialize and problem solve (eventually) in real time.
- Without gamma brainwave enhancement, I wouldn't have been able to take courses again.
- Without BioFlex Laser therapy, I wouldn't have experienced my heart rate dropping to the 80s from 130, my body temperature continue to normalize, and my brain relearn to perceive and walk with my new vision.
- Without Lindamood-Bell, I wouldn't have regained my reading comprehension and enjoy novels again, my second goal.
- Without home gamma audiovisual entrainment, I wouldn't have been able to keep pandemic anxiety down, restore energy consumed during the day, and stay focused on my goals.

- Without daily audiovisual entrainment at SMR/Beta, I wouldn't be able to calm my brain and boost energy, given the deep stressors I live with and complex, continuing PTSD.
- Without home BioFlex Laser, my pain and neuro-fatigue would ratchet up and heart rate variability drop again.

I no longer need strategies to concentrate, remember, talk, listen, watch a movie, read, write, take photographs, blog! And my brain continues to improve.

With each treatment, I regained some energy. Neuro-fatigue remains a problem, but I use energy conservation and am getting better at resting seven hours after I get up, as well as after a cognitive activity or exercise.

It's been a long road for me because I found and received these treatments years apart. I was also often at the forefront—I'm the case study that proves brain biofeedback's efficacy for brain injury. But today, it's possible to combine them into an effective treatment plan. Depending on your injury, you may only need weeks or months of treatments, although you may attend the clinic indefinitely for monitoring or maintenance visits, as life has a habit of throwing curveballs and having experts easily available makes them manageable. I find home devices essential as they're available anytime, including those difficult Friday nights and weekends.

Your Treatment Goal

- What do you want the most out of treating your neurons?
- What do you want to do without needing strategies or as few as necessary?

Write down here what you want:

_____

_____

_____

Yay!! Applaud yourself! I know. It sounds silly, clapping for yourself. But as I learnt from Prolifiko, applauding yourself helps you smile and boosts confidence.

Your Decision

Writing your treatment goal is you deciding on the next phase of your healing. The decision is to treat your neurons so you can establish a new, meaningful life. Without healing your brain, it is very hard to achieve your work, play, and social goals. This decision comprises three actions.

Action 1. Find a clinic that will use qEEG and evoke potentials to assess your brain activity. Alongside that, if you have trouble reading, find a Lindamood-Bell resource centre near you or one that provides virtual appointments. I contracted with their Australian resource centre so that I could attend virtually in the evenings. I also arranged for two-hour sessions, rather than the standard four-hour ones, because I lack at-home social support and my neuro-fatigue is too high to withstand four. I cleared my schedule of all other activities and built in rest time once the 81 hours of training was up.

Action 2. Attend prescribed treatments. These treatments will exhaust you, and you may not see results for a few weeks. But neurons don't heal without working the brain to the edge of its ability (see Principles of Treating the Brain later in this Step). Trusting the clinic or specialist helps endurance.

Action 3. Acquire and use, as prescribed, home devices such as Mind Alive audiovisual entrainment and/or cranioelectrical stimulation devices, and/or BioFlex Laser Therapy personal devices. I receive no remuneration for recommending these companies. Caring, innovative people founded these companies and continually improve their products to better meet the needs of their clients. I've had experience with both American-made and Canadian-made audiovisual entrainment devices, and the Canadian-researched and developed Mind Alive ones provide the best experience and a wide range of options.

Remember: spontaneous improvement continues after clinic treatment plans are completed.

Reach Out for Health Care That Treats Neurons and Heals Your Trauma and Grief

No one reached in to help me heal. The closest was in 2000 shortly after the car crash. The physiatrist who'd referred me to acupuncture to restore ulnar nerve function back in 1993 referred me to the psychologist he worked with. That took me so far, but for permanent regenerating and rewiring my neurons, I had to reach out.

I slowly began active searching in 2001. By 2005, after two years of 15 minutes of Googling per day for brain injury treatments, discovering none and switching to searching for ADD treatments, I found specialists who could possibly help. They were honest with me. I'd be a guinea pig. But having grown up knowing Judy Taylor, who'd prided herself on being a guinea pig for TPN, I had no problem with that.

reaching out for help means attending appointments consistently

This clinic and others I attended years later bent over backwards to help me. Like most with brain injury do, I developed close relationships with staff. Health care professionals and their staff may be the only ones happy to see us. Still, I learnt if I didn't show up for appointments, I received no help. I must always reach out and do the work.

Payment is an essential part of these relationships, whether by medicare, private insurance, or out of pocket. Our own initiative and persistence maintains them. It's difficult to grasp that when something like a pandemic happens and we can't attend appointments, we won't hear from them. It's a loss. Grief work helps soothe it.

The only one to reach in to me during the pandemic, without me reaching out first, was my orientation mobility trainer from the CNIB (Canadian National Institute for the Blind). It was part of their mandate, which medicare paid for.

Navigate Your Off Initiation Button to Reach Out

Brain injury often turns off our initiation button, or *Go Button*, as some call it. This is the ability to think about an activity and initiate it into action. After brain injury, we may think but cannot act. It isn't laziness or lack of motivation or malingering—it's a neurophysiological injury. When the injury is healed, the Go Button turns back on.

For well over a decade, my Go Button was off. Desperation to restore my brain drove me searching for treatments that would. My brain mattered a lot to me. Unconsciously powering that drive was the certainty that Jesus is glad I exist, that God is with me in my search, and God will show me the way. Yet I needed strategies to compensate for my neuro-fatigue and my off Go Button.

Routines

I set a routine of searching for 15 minutes per day on my computer. We work best with routines. What's your search-for-help routine? Can someone help you set up a routine to find a clinic that provides the diagnostics and neurostimulation treatments you need? Can you incorporate phone calls into your routine so that you can call clinics as part of that routine?

use phone notebooks to reach out →

I used phone notebooks. I learnt about phone notebooks from Dr. Claudia Osborn's book *Over My Head*. It works like this. Place a notebook beside every phone (or use your Notes app on your smartphone) to not only write down what people say but also, before you call someone, write out what you want to say. Writing it down means that when the inevitable voice mail answers, you'll know what to say by reading out loud the words in your phone notebook. Read these same words out loud if someone answers. I usually began my note with "Hello" followed by their name and my name. There's no shame in needing to write every word we'd say to start a phone conversation.

alarms and pacing makes reaching out possible →

Once I'd found a clinic, I set multiple alarms in my electronic calendar for appointments with colours to set them apart from my other scheduled tasks and events. I don't rely on post-its or paper calendars because when your Go Button is off, you need both sound and visuals to remind you.

Don't attend clinics that will berate you for being late or not set up a routine schedule for treatment appointments. Any health care professional who works with people with brain injury knows time is fluid in our minds until our neurons heal. To ensure we don't miss even one treatment, we need our appointments to be on the same day of the week at the same time.

Insist on it.

schedule rest 7 hours after you get up or before and after an appointment →

Schedule rest in your calendar for the hours and days before and after your treatments. Your brain worked hard, it's repairing itself, it needs all your energy after being stimulated into its repair work. Be like Nero Wolfe and don't let others interfere with your rest periods. You're not depressed. You're not unmotivated. Like a marathoner between training sessions whose muscles need rest in order to strengthen, you need to rest your brain to continue healing. And you need to persist through the debilitating neuro-fatigue. Neurons don't regrow and reconnect without intense, persistent work that's incredibly fatiguing, but which will ultimately improve your overall energy levels and dramatically increase function.

If you're lucky enough to have a person in your life who will drive you and is patient with your time issues, have them be ready to take you about 15 to 30 minutes before you have to leave because that's when they'll turn your Go Button on to get ready. Having a taxi regularly scheduled with the same driver could do the same thing. Otherwise, perhaps a bus schedule may help you get moving, like it does for me. Yes, it's stressful that you suddenly realize you're about to miss the bus, but at least it turns the Go Button on enough to get you going.

Remember: few reach in. So you have to use routines, pacing, and phone notebooks to reach out for treatments for your neurons.

Angst Is OK

When you find the right clinic and get a full diagnosis pinpointing which brain areas and neural networks are injured, and how they will restore your broken neurons, angst may follow the first rush of amazement and gratitude. Deep, deep grief may well up.

You may find angst building as you anticipate your first qEEG or, afterwards, when the clinic outlines your treatment plan of, for example, twice a week brain biofeedback plus home health care with audiovisual entrainment. This grief response to something so positive is normal. Don't listen to those who say you should feel good. Of course, you know this is a good thing. Of course, you know hope is coming to fruition. You've worked hard for it. But you've lived with unhealed brain injury for years without rehab or physicians offering you what's been available since you were first injured.

That's why the angst.

Seeing the coming treatment reminds you of the future taken from you. Instead of a future of healing that began right after your injury, you had a future of great suffering, of living in unimaginable hell. Then, to top it off, you had to fight for your brain. The fight has exhausted and scarred you.

when the fight is done, and the goal achieved, grief enters →

Return to Step Four to heal the grief.
But do not cancel your appointments.
Pursue your brain mapping and neurostimulation and/or neuromodulation treatments, even if after each one, you're exhausted and crying and feeling hopeless. I'm here to tell you that through two months of no change, the gruelling brain biofeedback appointments suddenly bore outstanding fruit. The work was worth it.

Use your home devices. My psychologist advised me audiovisual entrainment protocols can bring up subconscious emotions and thoughts, such as how much you've lost during the years without home treatments. Don't avoid using the devices; instead, allow yourself to feel the grief, maybe return to Step Four, but also set a small but effective goal as the reason to use your home device in the morning or at night. Goals can range from making old-fashioned oatmeal to blogging to better sleep. The goal will help you overcome avoiding the angst.

For example, you want to blog. You'll probably find the SMR/Beta audiovisual entrainment protocol helps you best with that. Use it a half hour before you've scheduled in your blog time. Allow yourself about ten minutes after the protocol ends to rest, drink water, and have a little cry. Then get up and go blog. Eventually, maybe weeks, maybe months, depending on your treatment progress and the extent of your injury, you'll not be crying or resting but getting up and blogging right away.

CHAPTER 27

NEUROSTIMULATION THERAPIES WORK

Diagnosis

Treating neurons begins with assessments that best suit our brain injury in order to prescribe individualized neurostimulation and neuromodulation therapies. These assessments are objective, not subjective, although questionnaires may support objective test findings.

To share knowledge about assessments that work for various brain injury types, and to inform about neurostimulation and neuromodulation therapies, I created the website Concussion Is Brain Injury based on my memoir of the same name. Before you continue here, skim the website to acquaint yourself with what's available to diagnose and treat your neurons.

LEARN MORE

Brain injury involves neurophysiological processes that I detail on *Brain Injury Is...* https://concussionisbraininjury.com/education/what-is-brain-injury/ and external effects https://concussionisbraininjury.com/education/.

Assessment Types

Each brain injury is unique. You may need only one kind of diagnostic assessment or multiple kinds. The ones that give the best picture of neuronal activity and dysfunction include qEEG, evoke potentials, SPECT, and DTI.

- QEEG creates a brain map of your brain's electrical activity. It separates out delta, theta, alpha, sensorimotor (SMR) rhythm, beta, gamma brainwaves, and muscle tension. This map shows the areas with inappropriate activity, for example, too much delta instead of beta; too little or too much coherence between brain areas; low power levels; neural network dysfunction. Thus, it gives the specialist a picture of what needs treating.
- Evoke Potentials includes qEEG brain maps, but also tests for visual and auditory startle responses within the brain versus to the outside world, processing speed, and cardiac function.
- SPECT scans use radioactive glucose to create a picture of which anatomical parts of the brain are using glucose, the brain's fuel, which reflects how active the brain is.
- Diffuse tensor imaging (DTI) uses MRI technology to provide a picture of your neural networks, to see which are damaged.

I've not found any clinic that does a comprehensive workup. I've had all these scans but the DTI (unavailable in my area) in different clinics.

Separately, my family physician ordered blood and urine tests; a physical trainer for elite athletes determined my exercise tolerance; some specialists assessed my balance crudely instead of with machinery; some assessed my pain levels on a scale of one to ten (which after a while I found irritating); several ordered sleep studies; neurorehab and insurance experts conducted IQ and neuropsychological tests (which I despise); and none collaborated.

You may have experienced similar.

No one specialist or clinic gathers a complete picture of your brain activity and function. Nor do clinics and specialists collaborate. Health care systems must fill this hole, sooner rather than later. Until then, we're on our own and have to be the connection between clinics and specialists. But knowing and finding the right kind of assessments you need is only the first step. The next is learning about effective treatments for brain injury.

LEARN MORE

Introduction to Diagnosis: https://concussionisbraininjury.com/diagnosis/introduction-to-diagnosis-of-brain-injury/

Diagnosis: https://concussionisbraininjury.com/diagnosis/

Thoughts on Effective Treatments

Effective treatments to heal brain injury include the following aspects:
- neurostimulation;
- supportive guidance by specialists;
- treatment goals;
- intense and frequent brain training;
- and objective testing before, during, and after to assess the extent of injury, individualize treatment, and measure progress towards our goals.

Specialists who treat brain injury to regain brain function and cognitions understand:
- the neurophysiological basis of brain injury;
- damaged neurophysiology needs to be treated;
- brains support brains, the phenomenon of a person in proximity to another enhancing the other's brain function and cognitions, whether that be reading, conversation, focusing, and so on;
- and listening and including the person are key so that their treatments will meet the person's goals as best as possible;
- and neurostimulation and neuromodulation harness the brain's neuroplasticity.

Although you may have heard the term "neuroplasticity," you may be unfamiliar with the innovative treatments that use the brain's electrical nature to speed up rewiring, repairing, and rebooting. Therapies that involve electricity create pictures of electroconvulsive therapy (ECT) and patients jerking on a hospital bed. The idea of one technology fitting brain injury of all types sounds fantastical, too.

Neither is true of neurostimulation and neuromodulation.

These technologies either harness the brain's regenerative capability so that the brain trains itself or use **battery-powered** direct electrical stimulation that allows a person to sit next to the specialist and engage in the activity they want to regain, for example, conversation. To use the pill analogy, neurostimulation is like a pill form; the individualized protocols are the prescribed ingredients in the pill; the electrodes or light array placements are the specific action of treatment. That's why it may seem like an unrealistic one-size-fits-all panacea, whereas it's in fact individualized medicine that works.

Unlike medications that flood the brain, neurostimulation and neuromodulation target specific locations and/or specific brainwaves to heal neurons permanently.

Photobiomodulation therapy (aka low-intensity laser therapy) has a systemic effect when placed on the back of the neck and brainstem regions. These light array placements enhance the body's ability to heal permanently instead of managing symptoms in the way medications do.

All these treatments may fatigue temporarily and lower blood pressure, requiring sitting quietly afterwards for a few minutes, but that's the extent of the side effects in my experience. As the treatments take effect, energy increases. Since they work the brain, replenishing brain fuel through food and water, as quickly as possible, is important.

Principles of Treating the Brain

Three principles guide most techniques of neurostimulation, neuromodulation, or brain training. Most take time to see results. Results last a few hours at first. They're usually permanent by the end of the treatment plan.

The First Principle. Reboot, repair, or rewire the brain.

The Second Principle. Train the brain to the edge of its ability through intensity and frequency of training over time with rest breaks. When training becomes easier, increase the difficulty so as to continue to train to the edge of ability. Reassess regularly through feedback and progress discussions with the client and by using the same objective assessments at the end of the treatment cycle as used for diagnosis. Exhaustion is a given, and so build in rest in between brain training sessions. Research shows learning works best with breaks in between.

The Third Principle. Engage in desired activity during or immediately after neurostimulation in order to stimulate rewiring of the neural networks involved in that activity.

LEARN MORE

"Medication is for symptom management. Medication does not cure. People with brain injury are looking for a cure or as close to one as current treatments can get." Go to https://concussionisbraininjury.com/treatments for information, research, and resources on neurostimulation therapies from brain biofeedback to audiovisual entrainment to photobiomodulation therapy and beyond.

CHAPTER 28

TREATING YOUR NEURONS

Action Plan: How Will You Get Appropriate Diagnostics and Treatments?

You know by now that you're worth treating your neurons and healing your trauma and grief. The only way to accomplish the former is by a clinic assessing your brainwave activity and cognitions using the diagnostic tests I discussed under Diagnosis, then treating your neurons with neurostimulation and neuromodulation.

But how to pursue this?
Try a big-picture **SMART** goal.
Specific
Measurable
Attainable
Relevant
Timely

Only you know your specific circumstances, what health care is available to you, what your financials are, what obstacles you face, and who is alongside versus resisting your drive to treat your neurons. Let's build your SMART goal.

Specific

For this Action Plan, sit at your computer or have your tablet with you in your quiet space. Open the website https://concussionisbraininjury.com and turn to a fresh page in your *Hello Healing* notebook and write at the top, "Action Plan for Healing My Brain." Then write your goal underneath, followed by your decision, "I want to regenerate my injured neurons."

Write below that "Specific. What I need to heal my neurons."

Go to https://concussionisbraininjury.com/diagnosis and copy the diagnostic tests you haven't received but need to get to know the full picture of your brain injury. Then click or tap on *Treatments*, and copy all the treatments you believe could help you.

You now have determined the specifics of your SMART goal.

Measurable

Write on a fresh page, "Measurable." How will you measure this goal? Break your goal down into measurable components. For example, the first step is researching the specific diagnostic tests and neurostimulation therapies you copied under "Specific." Review the research and testimonial pages for each therapy you copied in your notebook.

LEARN MORE

> See Mind Alive at https://mindalive.com for audiovisual entrainment and cranioelectrical stimulation.
> BioFlex Laser at https://bioflexlaser.com/ for photobiomodulation therapy.
> The ADD Centre at https://www.addcentre.com/ for brain biofeedback (neurofeedback).
> PoNS Therapy at https://ponstherapy.ca/ for Portable Neuromodulation Stimulator.
> Lindamood-Bell for visualizing and verbalizing reading comprehension retraining.

The next measurable step after research would be to find clinics and/or a Lindamood-Bell resource centre in your area (see the next Action Plan). A third measurable step would be to book an appointment for a qEEG or evoke potentials test. Or calling the nearest Lindamood-Bell resource centre to book an in-person or virtual reading comprehension assessment.

Another step would be to purchase one of the FDA- or Health Canada-approved audiovisual entrainment devices for home use. (Only ever purchase FDA and Health Canada approved medical devices.) As you work through each measurable goal, update your Measurable page with new or revised goals.

Attainable

Write on a fresh page, "Attainable." Use the decision-making tools under Action Plan: Developing Emotional Courage to determine how to attain each specific of this SMART goal. After deciding how to attain your goals, list them on a fresh page, one goal per line, with a short sentence on how you'll attain them. As you work through and attain each measurable goal, tick it off on this page.

Relevant and Timely

Relevant and Timely are a given. Treating your neurons is relevant because you have an injured brain and you want it treated. Timely is because you wanted this at the time of your injury, and what better time than now to make that happen at last?

Action Plan: Finding A Clinic

You're now ready to find a clinic that uses qEEG and evoke potentials tests, specifically the eVox System by Evoke Neuroscience. I wrote a section on my Concussion Is Brain Injury website on how to distinguish good help from bad and what questions to ask a prospective clinic. Begin by reading those resources at https://concussionisbraininjury.com/choices/ and https://concussionisbraininjury.com/choices/the-questions/.

Next, search on the internet for "qEEG mapping" and add your location. For example, I'd use the search term "qEEG mapping Toronto."

Or to find clinics who use Thought Technology systems, contact them at https://thoughttechnology.com/. Contact Evoke Neuroscience to find clinics that use their eVox system at https://evokeneuroscience.com/.

Contact only accredited specialists for brain mapping and brain biofeedback. The Biofeedback Certification International Alliance (https://www.bcia.org/) accredits specialists for HRV (heart rate variability) training and neurofeedback (brain biofeedback). You can search for accredited specialists at their website.

Clinics or specialists that diagnose also provide neurostimulation therapies. I recommend pairing their therapies with BioFlex Laser treatments at a clinic listed on their website. BioFlex Laser is photobiomodulation therapy that treats your brain and body systemically, improves HRV, and can enhance neurostimulation.

Home Devices

Home devices are essential. They provide the least expensive treatments, reduce stress, and enhance daily function. For home audiovisual entrainment and cranioelectrical devices, go to https://mindalive.com. They have testimonials, research, and other resources to help you decide on which product. I wrote about my experience with these home devices in *Concussion Is Brain Injury: Treating the Neurons and Me*, as well as on my blogs and *Psychology Today*.

You can either purchase a personal BioFlex Laser from https://bioflexlaser.com/ (under personal therapy systems) or at a BioFlex Laser clinic.

These companies update their standard protocols and devices. Some clinics can add prescribed treatments to your home devices.

Affording It

I don't know how I afforded all the treatments I've received over the years. Medicare covered only outpatient rehab and psychiatry. It covered community care for a few years until it cut funding. I paid for qEEG and evoke potentials tests using the eVox system and all neurostimulation and neuromodulation therapies. It cost me tens of thousands, yet my combined income sources are less than the poverty line. I don't think negotiation, cutting out clothes shopping, borrowing, paying back, parental support, borrowing again, cashing out some of my retirement savings, entirely accounts for how I did it. I believe two things were key for me:
1. I focused on my health as my top priority.
2. God helped me.

Money flows to what's important to us. Focusing on my health gave my money a destination and kept my non-health related spending to a minimum.

Powerful Minds

Even if you don't believe in God, I believe the power of focusing on your health above all else allows you to find a way. Our minds are powerful. Even stuck behind injured brains, when we focus our mind on treating our neurons, we can find our way there, though it seems impossible and improbable.

If we make work our priority instead of health, we inevitably fail, and we may worsen our injury. The same with socializing, hobbies, volunteering, or parenting. Ironically, we're more likely to get what we want when we pursue healing our brain injury.

when you focus on treating your neurons, work and play follow ➤

Without health, we cannot work, socialize, do a hobby, or parent—or we can only do those things in limited ways that require frustrating strategies. Focusing on our health—that is, healing our injured brain—means regaining those things we've lost as much as possible.

Funding

Despite my restricted circumstances, I've somehow funded diagnostics and treatments through negotiation, cycling through debt, cashing in some of my retirement savings, using every government support program I can, parental support, using credit cards to stave off payment for one month but always, always paying them off in full every month since the interest rates are ridiculous. No one method worked by itself. It was using the best combination for each circumstance that made it possible.

Rotary Clubs may help with acquiring home devices. They may also help pay for diagnosis and treatments at clinics. Compose a letter with your request. Include a supporting letter from your specialist if possible. Once you've proofread it, send it out to as many clubs in your region as you can find. Not all will reply. Those who do may take a few months to answer.

I've seen many try online funding drives, but I'm not sure how successful they are. I suspect people with supportive or extensive networks do better.

If you're flush with cash, why not set up a foundation to help those in poverty afford qEEG, Evoke Neuroscience's eVox System, and neurostimulation and neuromodulation therapies?

Action Plan: A Letter to Your Health Care Provider to Adopt Neurostimulation

I want to talk to health care professionals of all kinds—but especially your psychiatrists and neurologists—about why it's important for them to learn about neurostimulation treatments for brain injury. I'll use audiovisual entrainment (AVE) and cranioelectrical stimulation (CES) as examples about how learning this new field of medicine and adopting it in their practices will radically change their patients' lives. I used my Psychology Today posts on these two neurostimulation therapies as the basis for this letter.

Ask your treating physicians and other health care providers to treat your neurons and heal your brain. If they resist, copy the letter below and edit for your particular circumstance and SMART goal. Ask them to help you because Long Covid is a mass disabling event, and they'll also learn how to diagnose and treat those patients' neurophysiological dysfunction by helping you today.

To My Health Care Provider

I'm writing to you today about my brain injury and my desire to treat my neurons and heal my brain. I understand you're busy, but I believe it's worth learning about effective treatments to not only help me but also your patients with Long Covid and others with brain injury. It's a two-for-one benefit. You can add to your continuing education credits while learning how to help me regain my brain function and improve my quality of life significantly. I hope after reading this letter, you will help me diagnose and treat my brain injury in the same way cardiologists do heart disease or oncologists cancer.

Neurostimulation and neuromodulation dramatically improve brain function and, thus, their quality of life. Audiovisual entrainment (AVE) and cranioelectrical stimulation (CES) are the most accessible, portable, and affordable means of neurostimulation. With regular use, they will allow me to feel, to think clearer and easier, and to act or behave in line with who I am.

I share below one author's thoughts on why these effective technologies aren't being used widely after decades of research and clinical use: trust, overburden, and anxiety. I really, really want my brain healed as much as possible, far more than what I currently have. Medicine now has the research and clinical experience to make this happen. I hope you will consider these aspects of helping me achieve my goal of a better life.

Trust

The relationship between health care professional and patient or client determines outcome. Alliance and rapport foster trust; this trust leads to the person believing their health care professional knows what to do and following the instructions given to them. They're more likely to learn from therapy as well because trust will have created a willingness to pay attention. Trust will also encourage them to ask questions without fearing discharge because they asked or challenged their physician's opinions.

Trust requires time. A person will go into a relationship with societal trust: a doctor works to bring them back to health because that's what doctors do. A psychologist provides a caring atmosphere complete with couch. But personal trust from alliance and rapport, the kind that leads to the best outcomes, only develops through regular personal contact and from believing the professional listens and wants to do what it takes to help them achieve their treatment goals.

Unfortunately, experience teaches a person with brain injury that most professionals don't take the time to listen or align themselves with the healing they crave. And so when, for example, the trusted social worker suggests seeing an unknown psychologist for neurostimulation, the person balks because they doubt this unknown psychologist will be trustworthy. Neurostimulation sounds woo-woo and potentially like ECT, not a prescription we want to receive from a new, unknown health care professional. Receiving neurostimulation and/or neuromodulation therapy from the trusted social worker, though, fosters assent. But if they don't trust their social worker, either, they'll find any excuse not to agree.

Burden

Brain injury requires seeing multiple specialists. Getting health care becomes a job of juggling appointments and prescriptions that range from exercises to daily activities of living to taking medications that don't work well. One-off consultant appointments interfere with regular appointments that keep us going. It's frustrating and despairing. And so when a psychiatrist, for example, suggests seeking neurostimulation with a psychologist, the person balks. It's one more regular appointment to add on to the already onerous health care schedule. The psychiatrist providing it themself means it's physically doable for the person in their weekly life.

Anxiety

Because few have heard of neurostimulation, never mind understand what it is, the thought of using it creates anxiety. We all know about medications because we've been brought up with pills—acetylsalicylic acid for a headache, acetaminophen for fevers, vitamins, and minerals. Taking a prescribed medication may create anxiety around the prescription's effects, but not in the pill itself.

But that's not true for neurostimulation.

Not only would the prescription cause anxiety but also the technique as well. Thoughts revolve: *What does it look like? What will it feel like? How do you use it?*

It's not as easy as swallowing a pill. You have to choose the right protocol, remember to drink water, know how to put on the eyesets and headphones (stressful when even brushing teeth is difficult), and so on. A person with anxiety, including anxiety from brain injury, will become so anxious at the thought of this unknown technique, they'll balk. Read more about why anxiety after brain injury is a physical manifestation of the injury at https://concussionisbraininjury.com/education.

The only way to overcome anxiety at trying a new technique is by their health care professional doing it in office as part of their regular appointment. Their trusted professional next to them comforts and alleviates anxiety, which leads to assent. In addition, by walking them through the protocols, asking how they feel and what they see, teaching which protocol they're using and perhaps why, the professional helps them transition to using this novel technique at home.

For the reasons of trust, not overburdening with appointments, and overcoming anxiety, every health care professional ought to learn about and use AVE and CES in office and guide at-home use. Also, using AVE and CES during a talk therapy session can relax a person so that they talk more easily.

AVE and CES are only the easiest and most affordable neurostimulation treatments. Others, used in clinic, by trained and certified professionals, effect permanent treatment. You can learn more about the various kinds at https://concussionisbraininjury.com/treatments.

Please consider using neurostimulation in my regular appointments with you and find and work with a clinic that provides qEEG, the eVox system, and neurostimulation therapies to radically improve my life.

CHAPTER 29

STRETCHING YOUR CONNECTIONS

"Gertie asserted that all she did in our phone calls was listen to me. *How could I remember the details of her last day in our last phone call so many months ago if I was the only one talking? How could I recall those details when I'd forget important events like the day of a birthday?* I dragged in breath and tuned back in. 'I heard little empathy from you for me. You cannot just listen. You always give forceful responses, and you get offended if we don't take it.'"

From Concussion Is Brain Injury: Treating the Neurons and Me.

Empathy

Outwardly, people see no empathy in us. Inwardly, we care deeply about others. We worry over the stress we see in our spouse or mother. We desperately want to connect with friends, siblings, children—help them, laugh with them, listen to them. But we can't break through the barriers our brain injury has thrown up. Our broken cognitions, freaky memory lapses, and fragmented communication abilities create challenging obstacles; neuro-fatigue makes getting out of bed an ordeal. How then can we express empathy?

When loved ones' and specialists' ideation of us is we have no empathy, we can listen and commiserate all we want, but they won't remember our empathy.

other people with brain injury see your empathy

Can we express our empathy, and have the energy to do so, in the way others can see?

I've learnt there's not much we can do when loved ones fib we lack empathy and convince our specialists of it, the ones who adhere to DSM categories over qEEG, evoke potentials, SPECT, and DTI.

Instead of fighting their falsehood about you lacking empathy, turn your attention to those who recognize and need your empathy, including others with brain injury. They see the truth and will value your empathy, however challenged you are in showing it. They'll roll with how you express it in all your brain injury glory, for they know how hard it is to express through brain injury barriers and what you truly feel inside.

Effective Treatments Break Down Communication Barriers

As neurostimulation and/or neuromodulation reboot microglia and repair and rewire neurons, the parts of your brain that feel and communicate empathy will come back online. You'll find it easier to perceive and express empathy. Trauma breaking your trust in others may complicate this restoration. In this case, a comprehensive approach that includes a psychiatrist or psychologist providing trauma therapy concurrently with neurostimulation appointments will help. Alternatively, use audiovisual entrainment, cranioelectrical stimulation, or photobiomodulation therapy home devices prior to social engagements so that you have more energy, clearer thinking, and more accessible emotions to perceive and express empathy even when you expect no reciprocal empathy and trusting others eludes you.

Take heart that I continue to heal despite my lack of trust in others and my contradictory trust in God. I'm certain God helps me; yet I distrust my future and whatever seemingly good things the Holy Spirit nudges me towards. As Maude Barlow wrote in her 2022 book *Still Hopeful*, "Despair can be countered by action." Hope arrives when we act.

My experience these past 22 years and the effect of intergenerational trauma decimated my ability to trust, yet I didn't let go of my childhood decision to be a trustable, empathetic listener. Hold on to your integrity, remain on your lifelong healing path, and you will see progress.

Action Plan: Reaching Out to Others

One of the best ways to help you feel better when the pain of life takes you over is to reach out to others on social media having a hard time and validating their experience or giving them a boost. When we connect with others and support them, our neurons release oxytocin, which gives us a good feeling. See Mirror Neurons and Oxytocin under Step One: Loved and Unloved.

Encouraging others gives you more than a hit of oxytocin; it also tells you, you matter in this world. You have something to give; there are people out there who appreciate your generosity and your person. This action of reaching out to boost another counters the judgements, labelling, criticism, and ostracization you've suffered unjustly for so long.

Support Others Within the Boundaries of Your Neuro-Fatigue

The advantage of reaching out on social media is you can do it within your neuro-fatigue limitations, when the need arises in you, not only at a scheduled brain injury community meeting or social event. Twitter is easier because it's short; it doesn't strain your attention span or reading comprehension as much as social media with longer comment spaces do. You type and send. It's that easy.

In real life, you can reach out to the person who sits beside you on a park bench, or looks confused as they stare at a public transit map.

Sometimes, you won't want to talk to anybody, and that's OK. But when you want to rid yourself of the pain rising in you, and you feel you can say, "Hello?" try it.

The only caveat is don't approach people who look angry or grim. Keep yourself safe because your brain injury renders you vulnerable. It's a bit of a paradox, I find—the injury that makes me a sitting duck also makes me impervious to the danger. That's when I need to try and call on my intellect and my habit of taking my time to assess before acting.

Most humans respond with gratitude and relief when someone reaches out to them. And maybe because it doesn't happen often for you, doing that for another makes it sweeter.

Action Plan: Meaning in Life

I wrote earlier about the Positive Psychology **Optimism Test** and the **VIA Survey of Character Strengths**.

Another questionnaire I found helpful, to validate my state of mind, was the **Meaning in Life Questionnaire**. Go to https://authentichappiness.org and click or tap Questionnaires. You'll find this one near the bottom of the list in the section *Meaning Questionnaires*.

heal your neurons before taking mood questionnaires →

I didn't take any of the mood questionnaires because brain injury mimics mood and emotion issues. These questionnaires probably don't include in their research injury to the brain's emotion centres or how microglia dysfunction affects mood. For mood and emotions, it's better to first work on healing your brain. Sadness, grief, lack of motivation, no initiation are all natural outflows of the brain injury and its consequences. Heal the injury and you go a long way towards healing them.

God

For those who believe in God, meaning encompasses having faith that God exists, is there for us, and will work with us to reach our dreams, to return to health, and to be in mithra. To fulfill your mithra needs, when you look for a church or synagogue or temple, look for an inclusive one. Exclusion hurt you, prevented you from healing, and separated you from mithra; so don't carry exclusionary thinking into how you relate to God and who you worship with. All of us are God's children. God loves all of us. To exclude anyone, or label anyone, for whatever reason works against God's love and against mithra.

Nature

You don't need to believe in God or a Creator or Higher Power to find meaning in life. Knowing you're part of the planet and the universe generates awe and a sense of connection with every atom that makes up this wondrous material existence. As such, your life is necessary for the universe and so has meaning.

As the cosmos created us, so too did it create other humans and species. It's one thing to be excluded and to live apart from others in order to focus on healing ourselves, it's another to work to exclude certain people from ours and others' lives. Don't do to them what they did to you—it diminishes who you are and prevents growth—but wait for them as I discussed in Forgiveness Is Not Reconciliation in Step Two: Relationships. Instead, find resources to help you fulfill your mithra needs with a supportive group of people, including online communities.

Reflecting on the Questionnaire Results

Read the results of the Meaning in Life Questionnaire, then file them away in your *Hello Healing* notebook for a few days. You know how long you take to process information or absorb new knowledge. Take the results out when that time has elapsed and consider each result.

What do your Meaning in Life results tell you about yourself?

Write your thoughts in your notebook and reward yourself when done for the day. Repeat as necessary until you feel you've fully processed the results.

If you struggle with your meaning in life, ask yourself (and write out) what will help you take the first step towards having a purpose or feeling you mean something?

Action Plan: Fun

What is fun for you?

In your *Hello Healing* notebook, turn to a fresh page and write at the top, "What I find fun." Underline the word, "I."

Then list everything you find fun. Not what others tell you or what they think you should do with them for fun. Don't list what you used to think was fun *before* your brain injury—list what you like *now*. Some examples:

- Sleeping in.
- Watching a movie in the afternoon.
- You and your dog lazing on the couch.
- Walking empty streets when people are at work.
- Reading trashy novels all day long.
- Having coffee with one friend in the middle of the day.
- Baking.
- Cooking your favourite dishes or your spouse's favourite dishes.
- Hand wrestling with your cat.
- Blogging or tweeting or taking photos or painting.
- Gardening for 10 minutes a day.

You get the idea. Fun things don't have to involve other people nor conform to their idea of length. Since you're alone, you need to have fun on your own to diminish the feeling of loss. This also means you can have fun when your neuro-fatigue and schedule allow. You don't have to worry about others' convenience conflicting with your energy levels and diminishing your enjoyment.

If you're fortunate to have a friend or family member who likes to do things with you your way, include that in your list.

Once you have your fun list, choose the one that calls out to you right now and do it. Then reward yourself.

Rewarding yourself for having fun pumps you up, builds self-worth, increases the likelihood you'll do what you find fun again. Brain injury becomes such a slog, recovery a soul-sucking job, that having fun our way vanishes. Rewarding yourself for daring to have fun your way tells you it's good.

Check your fun list daily and choose one item to do that day. As you discover new things, add to it. Since habits have a habit of vanishing, schedule checking your fun list or use an alarm app to remind you. Don't schedule an audible alarm every day because alarm fatigue will set in and irritate you. Instead, schedule frequently enough so you remember to have fun most days without your alarm annoying you.

Treating My Neurons and Healing Myself Have Given Me...

I went from confused, extremely reduced cognitive functioning, to regaining most of my talents. Although I still struggle with neuro-fatigue, exhaustion, stamina, and other brain injury manifestations that prevent me from working or socializing like a non-injured person, the list of radical improvements is extensive. You can read about them in my memoir or blog. I write a few thoughts here.

Brain Injury Is Like an Earthquake

Earthquakes are part of our planet's life cycle. We float on Earth's tectonic plates, which occasionally crash or dive underneath each other. The plates' crashing brings nutrients to the surface, and what's destructive becomes constructive. Smaller quakes follow a sudden, large, jarring quake as the plates settle into a new pattern. But when humans build poorly, congregate around the seams, many die and the earthquake's constructive effect gets lost in the human-enhanced destruction.

Brain injury is like an earthquake. Why does it happen? Like Job, we may never know. Like me, you may never be thankful for it. But it happened, and an understandable lack of gratitude doesn't have to stop reconstruction nor settling into new patterns.

We learn about earthquakes from seismologists, high school teachers, and people who've lived through them and gained wisdom on how to survive and thrive. We don't individually relearn what experts and wise elders have learned; instead, we learn from them and use their knowledge to protect ourselves from harm. That's the advantage of humanity's social biology: collectively we know more than individually.

Similarly, we learn about brain injury from others. It's impossible for every injured person to gain neurophysiological, psychological, physiological, and experiential knowledge individually. Instead, we learn from others and use gained wisdom and knowledge to protect ourselves from the cascading damage that flows out from the original injury. Or when standard medical care has failed us, to use their experiences as a guide to our healing.

The Future

When the past has trashed your health and life, when even yesterday often contains strife, thinking about the future becomes scary. So don't. Thinking about today is enough. With brain injury, daily life comprises daily struggles from being able to make meals before your stomach screams at you from unrecognized hunger, to being able to make it to an appointment on time, to sleepiness and neuro-fatigue crashing you onto the couch. So don't burden yourself with forcing positive thoughts about the future. Instead, use your brain injury's propensity to stay in the present moment; make the present moment what you want, as much as you're able to.

  Right now, as you read this book, you're in the present while affecting your future without making yourself think positively about it or devising plans for it. The only thought you need is to take a step in the present that'll wend your way to a better future is how to treat your neurons and heal your trauma and grief. Taking one step at a time is action that leads to hope.

Using Modern Medicine to Get Up and Going

I wake up, and within seconds, psychic pain squeezes my heart. I resist, make myself slide on my CES's ear clips, and turn it to the intensity that best helps me. Within six minutes, the stimulation pries psychic pain's fingers off my heart. I'll spend an hour with it on, as well as the audiovisual entrainment SMR/Beta protocol, while either dozing or strolling through Twitter. I'm then able to get up and hit my keyboard running, with some coffee, of course. Or I pick up the latest novel I'm reading and settle in to enjoy it.

  The point is, you don't need positive thinking about the future to get going in the morning. And you don't need a health care professional to learn about neurostimulation and start treating you in order to discover its benefits. You have the power to grab what modern medicine can give you in your own home. Many have now come before you and written about their experiences, experiences that can reassure and teach you; thousands of studies have proven at-home neurostimulation's efficacy. These devices may not permanently heal your neurons, and you'll need to learn which protocols work best for you, but it'll help you get up and going today. And today is the only thing that matters when you're living with the devastating effects of brain injury.

Healing the Brain Means Learning to Live With More Control Over Yourself

After years of living with no control over my brain, I gradually regained control over my thoughts and emotions. A cognition can heal suddenly or can flicker on and off, then suddenly and dramatically be fully better. Spontaneous healing continues after in-clinic neurostimulation therapies end, which may be subtle at first but dramatic over time. Sometimes improvements confuse. But after you process the latest amazing change, you'll realize that you've regained some control over a cognition or function. While control comes with treating your neurons, responsibility for retaining and strengthening that control is part of personal growth. It's a process, so forgive yourself when you stumble. Remind yourself that you now have the power through healed neurons to keep improving control where it returns while retaining your post-injury gifts and lessons.

Healing What Matters the Most

What mattered most to me was my reading. Through 18 years of looking for help, trying every method offered to me, quitting, despairing, trying again, I didn't think I'd ever really give up on my goal of reading books again. But I did. And that's when I was told about Lindamood-Bell's reading assessment and underwent their visualizing and verbalizing program. I regained my reading comprehension for novels, neuroscience, and philosophy of mind. But that was only the first step. The next was daily practice to reinforce my regained brain function and to expand it. Concurrently with daily practice, I worked on recovering emotionally and processing my reading loss grief.

you have a choice to make: continuing as you are or healing your brain and yourself →

Joy is not about *feeling* happy; it's about seeing beauty and the good, taking the next step in healing in the midst of raw pain and despair.

Continuing as you are is like the adage of doing the same thing over and over while expecting a different outcome. When you choose the demanding path to heal your brain and yourself, you never know when waning hope will change into a rewarding reality. It's OK to cry as you tread this path as long as you don't turn your back on the opportunity to treat your neurons and heal your trauma and grief. Eventually, your crying will turn into a new way of living, one that contains joy.

I pray for you much strength, emotional courage, and hope as you embark on this new path of healing.

READINGS

Don't Forgive Too Soon
Extending the Two Hands That Heal
Dennis Linn, Sheila Fabricant Linn, Matthew Linn
This 1997 book uses humorous illustrations, accessible text, and personal openness to help readers understand and learn to forgive without the usual wagging-finger judgement. Two of the authors were or are Jesuit priests; the third is the wife of one. The Linns filled this accessible book with illustrative stories and practical exercises. They also provide real-world examples.

The Gathas of Zarathushtra
Hymns in Praise of Wisdom
Illustrated and divided into sections, this small 1999 book contains the surviving ancient Gathas, translated into English along with research-backed commentary by Piloo Nanavutty.

Over My Head
A Doctor's Own Story of Head Injury from the Inside Looking Out
Claudia L. Osborn
Locked inside a brain-injured head looking out at a challenging world is the premise of this extraordinary year 2000 autobiography. *Over My Head* is an inspiring story of how one woman comes to terms with the loss of her identity and the courageous steps (and hilarious missteps) she takes while learning to rebuild her life.

Lifeliner
The Judy Taylor Story
Shireen Jeejeebhoy
My 2007 biography on Judy Taylor, the first person in the world to live without eating. This book chronicles the development of home total parenteral nutrition from the patient's point of view and looks at how she thrived after the catastrophic, sudden loss of all her bowels. Physicians on the international stage bought it to enhance their patient care.

The Job Sessions
Why Do The Innocent Suffer?
Shireen Jeejeebhoy
An ebook with handouts on the *Book of Job* in the Old Testament of the Bible. Considered one of the bible's oldest books, it's both prose and poetry about how a successful, wealthy man suffers unexplainable, unjust misfortune and his way back to a full life.

Concussion Is Brain Injury
Shireen Jeejeebhoy
A collection of my blog posts from between 2009 and 2012 on my brain injury, challenges that arise in care and trying to return to normal life, and learning how to heal from it.

Concussion Is Brain Injury
Treating the Neurons and Me (Revised Edition)
Shireen Jeejeebhoy
Revised, updated, and written in narrative form with separate Learnings sections, my 2017 memoir brings to life the experience of trying to recover from brain injury. I divided it into sections reflecting the various stages of my recovery. Each narrative section concludes with the learnings from that time period to provide the reader knowledge and practical understanding of how to treat injured neurons.

Surprised By Hope
Rethinking Heaven, the Resurrection, and the Mission of the Church
NT Wright
Written by British first-century scholar and Christian bishop Wright, this 2014 book upends our understandings of the New Testament. Through his scholarship, Wright shows how the centuries and changing cultures have distorted our translations and understandings. He challenges our 21st century assumptions about the meanings of Jesus's resurrection and provides a different concept of hope.

How To Hold A Grudge
From Resentment to Contentment—the Power of Grudges to Transform Your Life
Sophie Hannah

This 2018 book by the best-selling novelist provides a practical way to process grudges and gets rid of blame and judgement around them. The writing is conversational and humorous.

The Angel and the Assassin
The Tiny Brain Cell That Changed the Course of Medicine
Donna Jackson Nakazawa
Written in accessible neuroscience, this 2021 book chronicles the author's journey back to health and the reason why she pursued trying to understand the neuroscience behind her condition. It centres on her investigation into the research being done on microglia and what that means for people with mental illness and brain injury. The sub-title is deceptive because so far medicine hasn't changed its course, but hopefully this research and its clinical applications will do so.

What Happened To You?
Conversations on Trauma, Resilience, and Healing
Bruce D. Perry and Oprah Winfrey
This beautifully designed 2021 book is written as a conversation between Perry and Oprah. Each of the 10 chapters begins with personal reflections by each author, and then dives into the research and science behind what trauma is and the effect of trauma on the brain, behaviour, and perspective of the world. The design is not all that accessible. I found the italics very hard to read, and the beautiful blue text in the hardcover doesn't have enough contrast for the visually impaired. However, if you can persevere through those bad design choices, this book provides a ton of understanding. Diagrams help the process.

The Grieving Brain
The Surprising Science of How We Learn from Love and Loss
Mary-Frances O'Connor
A fascinating 2022 book by Associate Professor of Psychology O'Connor. The writing is easy on the brain, which is good since the topic is emotionally difficult and O'Connor covers many research studies on grief and grieving. She uses diagrams to illustrate some new concepts around grief.

Still Hopeful
Lessons from a Lifetime of Activism
Maude Barlow
In this timely 2022 book, Barlow counters the prevailing atmosphere of pessimism that surrounds us and offers lessons of hope that she has learned from a lifetime of activism.

Websites

Psychology Today: Concussion Is Brain Injury https://www.psychologytoday.com/ca/blog/concussion-is-brain-injury

Concussion Is Brain Injury website https://concussionisbraininjury.com

Each of the websites below have pages on the research behind their neurostimulation and neuromodulation technology. I've personally used and healed from their treatments and devices and am not benefitting in any way financially from mentioning them here or in the book. I'm not directly connecting to their research pages because companies have a habit of changing their page URLs. You can also find explanations and research links on these and more under https://concussionisbraininjury.com/treatments/.

Mind Alive, Inc. https://mindalive.com

The ADD Centre https://addcentre.com

BioFlex Laser https://bioflexlaser.com/

Thank You

Thank you for reading this book.

If you found it helpful, please encourage your friends, family, associates, neighbours, heck, anyone, to buy a copy or request a copy at their library so that they can heal from it, too!

Find more information at https://jeejeebhoy.ca
or at https://concussionisbraininjury.ca

* * *

ACKNOWLEDGEMENTS

This book appeared like one of my novels—unbidden. Usually, my non-fiction books arise from thought, from conversations with another person, not as an idea suddenly appearing in my mind. Although I didn't think of myself as a person who could write self-help, the idea excited me. I didn't talk about it at first as I mulled it over. Then an urge gripped me that I must write it now. To me, an urge that grips me, that crescendos in my mind until I must obey, are like urgent messages from God. I'm not saying that God demanded I write this book. It's more like it was something I had to do; I'd only find out the reason as I did it and after it was done.

I received immediate validation from Bec Evans, one of the co-founders along with Chris Smith of Prolifiko, and the Prolifiko writing community, that this was a book worth writing.

I became interested in Prolifiko when it was first launched. I tried out some of their offerings for awhile. But when I heard about their 7-day writing sprints, I leapt in. I didn't expect it to become an integral part of my writing life. Seven days suits my brain-injury temperament, and it's resulted in me finishing a few manuscripts. What I didn't expect was the comfortable and rewarding writing community that organically grew around these sprints. I dedicated this book to the Prolifiko writing community for their encouragement, external motivation, and feeling of solidarity in this hard, lonely, exciting writing life. They gave me a sense of normalcy and escape from brain injury.

I'll always be grateful to Bec and Chris for generously providing us with their writing sprints and the innumerable practical encouragements they gave me. I want to thank Bec as well for her feedback on my title and cover. I learnt from her what makes a good title and aspects of good cover design.

When I realized I was going to write this book, I asked my Tweeps what they would look for in such a book. I want to thank Aurelia Cotta, Kelly Boreson, Donald Nicolson (who also wrote the Foreword to my revised memoir), Bill MacDonald, Anne Ricketts, Keith Isley, and Michelle Munt for their feedback, support, encouragement, lively conversations, and illuminating tweets over the years. Your presences in my life are invaluable to me. Without learning from you, I would not have felt motivated to keep writing about brain injury.

Acknowledgements

I've had various health care professionals over the years who've supported my writing, all of whom I'm grateful to, but there are two who stand out for this book. I miss my behavioural therapist Lisa Lariviere. Before we had to part ways several years ago, she alone made sure I kept writing novels and publishing them. She used my strengths and buttressed my weaknesses to keep me functional and on track. Her lessons guide me to this day, including those I struggle or fail to maintain without her practical presence. Lisa read all my books while working with me, and I cannot tell you how much that meant to me. When she talked about them, I knew it came from an honest, knowledgeable place. There's a big difference between someone who says, "I support you and you're a good writer," without reading one of your books, or only a few pages here and there, and someone who has read them. The latter provides true support and validation that boosts self-confidence. So it is with Dr. Michael Zitney as well, whose interest in both my memoir and this book spur me on today. Thank you, Lisa and Michael!!

I'm grateful to Greg Ioannou and Greg's 2022 editing intern Clarisse Smith for chewing over the idea of mithra and brainstorming with me a new term for it. Clarisse's feedback on the first part of my manuscript clarified some issues I needed to address in how people perceive brain injury symptoms. Greg has been with me since I first began working on *Lifeliner*, and I've learnt much from him over the years. I'm thankful for his generous gift of time and thought.

Every book is not possible without my mother. Mum (spelled with a "u"!) began teaching me to read before my first memory, around about 18 months or younger. She introduced me to the wondrous entity called a "library." And modelled voracious reading. As if that wasn't a big enough gift, Mum buys my books, talks up my books, gives them away (hoping the recipients will buy more), occasionally is critical, which keeps me thinking. If Mum starts talking with you about one of my novels or non-fiction books, you're going to end up buying it! But most of all, like many mothers everywhere, she makes my life possible. Thank you seems inadequate. But thank you, Mum!!!

www.ingramcontent.com/pod-product-compliance
Lightning Source LLC
Chambersburg PA
CBHW020135130526
44590CB00039B/184